Current Concepts in the Treatment of the Rheumatoid Hand, Wrist and Elbow

Guest Editor

KEVIN C. CHUNG, MD, MS

HAND CLINICS

www.hand.theclinics.com

February 2011 • Volume 27 • Number 1

SAUNDERS an imprint of ELSEVIER, Inc.

W.B. SAUNDERS COMPANY
A Division of Elsevier Inc.

1600 John F. Kennedy Blvd. • Suite 1800 • Philadelphia, Pennsylvania 19103

http://www.theclinics.com

HAND CLINICS Volume 27, Number 1
February 2011 ISSN 0749-0712, ISBN-13: 978-1-4557-0455-2

Editor: Debora Dellapena

Hand Clinics (ISSN 0749-0712) is published quarterly by Elsevier Inc., 360 Park Avenue South, New York, NY 10010-1710. Months of publication are February, May, August, and November. Business and Editorial Offices: 1600 John F. Kennedy Blvd., Ste. 1800, Philadelphia, PA 19103-2899. Customer Service Office: 3251 Riverport Lane, Maryland Heights, MO 63043. Periodicals postage paid at New York, NY and at additional mailing offices. Subscription price is $338.00 per year (domestic individuals), $540.00 per year (domestic institutions), $169.00 per year (domestic students/residents), $385.00 per year (Canadian individuals), $617.00 per year (Canadian institutions), $459.00 per year (international individuals), $617.00 per year (international institutions), and $223.00 per year (international and Canadian students/residents). Foreign air speed delivery is included in all *Clinics* subscription prices. All prices are subject to change without notice. **POSTMASTER:** Send address changes to *Hand Clinics*, Elsevier Health Sciences Division, Subscription Customer Service, 3251 Riverport Lane, Maryland Heights, MO 63043. Customer Service (orders, claims, online, change of address): Elsevier Health Sciences Division, Subscription Customer Service, 3251 Riverport Lane, Maryland Heights, MO 63043. Tel: 1-800-654-2452 (U.S. and Canada); 314-447-8871 (outside U.S. and Canada). Fax: 314-447-8029. E-mail: journalscustomerservice-usa@elsevier.com (for print support); journalsonlinesupport-usa@elsevier.com (for online support).

Reprints. For copies of 100 or more of articles in this publication, please contact the Commercial Reprints Department, Elsevier Inc., 360 Park Avenue South, New York, New York 10010-1710. Tel.: 212-633-3812; Fax: 212-462-1935; E-mail: reprints@elsevier.com.

Hand Clinics is covered in *MEDLINE/PubMed (Index Medicus)*, *Current Contents/Clinical Medicine*, *EMBASE/Excerpta Medica*, and *ISI/BIOMED*.

Printed and bound by CPI Group (UK) Ltd, Croydon, CR0 4YY

Transferred to Digital Print 2011

Contributors

GUEST EDITOR

KEVIN C. CHUNG, MD, MS
Professor of Surgery, Section of Plastic Surgery, Department of Surgery, Assistant Dean for Faculty Affairs, University of Michigan Medical School, Ann Arbor, Michigan

AUTHORS

RONALD J. ANDERSON, MD
Division of Rheumatology, Immunology and Allergy, Brigham and Women's Hospital; Associate Professor of Medicine, Harvard Medical School, Boston, Massachusetts

PHILIP E. BLAZAR, MD
Assistant Professor, Hand/Upper Extremity Service, Department of Orthopaedic Surgery, Brigham and Women's Hospital, Harvard Medical School, Boston, Massachusetts

FRANK D. BURKE, MBBS, FRCS
Professor of Hand Surgery, Pulvertaft Hand Centre, Royal Derby Hospital, Derby, United Kingdom

KEVIN C. CHUNG, MD, MS
Professor of Surgery, Section of Plastic Surgery, Department of Surgery, Assistant Dean for Faculty Affairs, University of Michigan Medical School, Ann Arbor, Michigan

PHILIP J. CLAPHAM, BS
Research Assistant, Section of Plastic Surgery, University of Michigan Health System, Ann Arbor, Michigan

WILLIAM P. COONEY III, MD
Professor Emeritus, Department of Orthopedic Surgery, Mayo Clinic, Rochester, Minnesota; Pro-sports, Hand and Upper Extremity, Vero Beach, Florida

GEORGE S.M. DYER, MD
Clinical Instructor in Orthopaedic Surgery, Harvard Medical School; Chief of Hand and Upper Extremity Surgery, VA Boston Healthcare; and Staff Physician, Department of Orthopaedic Surgery, Brigham and Women's Hospital, Boston, Massachusetts

POUYA ENTEZAMI, BS
Research Assistant, Section of Plastic Surgery, University of Michigan Health System, Ann Arbor, Michigan

DAVID A. FOX, MD
Professor of Internal Medicine, Division Chief of Rheumatology, University of Michigan Medical School, Ann Arbor, Michigan

DANIEL B. HERREN, MD
Head, Department of Upper Extremity and Handsurgery, Schulthess Clinic, Zurich, Switzerland

J. MICHELLE KAHLENBERG, MD, PhD
Fellow, Division of Rheumatology, University of Michigan, Ann Arbor, Michigan

JEFFREY H. KOZLOW, MD
Resident Physician, Section of Plastic Surgery, Department of Surgery, University of Michigan Health System, Ann Arbor, Michigan

PETER M. MURRAY, MD
Professor of Orthopaedic Surgery, Consultant in Hand and Microvascular Surgery, Department of Orthopedic Surgery, Mayo Clinic, Jacksonville, Florida

MARCO RIZZO, MD
Associate Professor, Department
of Orthopedic Surgery, Mayo Clinic,
Rochester, Minnesota

STEPHAN F. SCHINDELE, MD
Consultant, Department of Upper Extremity
and Handsurgery, Schulthess Clinic, Zurich,
Switzerland

SANDEEP J. SEBASTIN, MCh
Associate Consultant, Department of Hand
and Reconstructive Microsurgery, National
University Health System, Singapore

BEAT R. SIMMEN, MD
Senior Consultant, Department of Upper
Extremity and Handsurgery, Schulthess
Clinic, Zurich, Switzerland

BARRY P. SIMMONS, MD
Associate Professor of Orthopaedic Surgery;
Chief of Hand and Upper Extremity Service,
Department of Orthopaedic Surgery,
Brigham and Women's Hospital, Boston,
Massachusetts

JENNIFER F. WALJEE, MD, MS
House Officer, Section of Plastic Surgery,
Department of Surgery, University
of Michigan Health System, Ann Arbor,
Michigan

E.F. SHAW WILGIS, MD
Director of Research, The Curtis National Hand
Center, Union Memorial Hospital, Baltimore,
Maryland

Contents

Contributions of historical analyses to the development of a cogent etiologic theory of rheumatoid arthritis (RA) have been limited to date. In this article, the authors analyze this literature with respect to the types and conclusions of the research that has been conducted, present the major points of evidence and conclusions that have been drawn, and trace the evolution of 3 historical theories of RA. The authors combine a comprehensive overview of paintings and paleopathological investigations with consideration of contemporary immunologic and genetic studies.

Over the past 2 decades, the treatment of rheumatoid arthritis (RA) has been revolutionized by advances in the understanding of its pathologic mechanisms and the development of drugs that target them. These newer medications have shown great promise at improving disease outcomes, but they come with notable side effects that can pose long-term treatment challenges and difficulties in the perioperative arena. In this article, the major manifestations of RA and the current medical options for management are discussed. Complications from treatment are then reviewed, and special consideration is given to perioperative medication recommendations.

The clinical picture of rheumatoid arthritis (RA) is best viewed as a combination of systemic symptoms associated with the inflammatory process and articular symptoms related both to potentially reversible synovitis and structural damage brought on by inflammation. In simple terms, the treatment of inflammation is medical, and structural lesions often require surgical solutions. The prime indications for surgery in patients with RA are essentially determined by the patient and consist of a desire to obtain pain relief and/or functional improvement. Pain is difficult to quantify. Essential concepts regarding surgical intervention are that surgery is elective in all but a few rare situations and always requires local therapy. Any evaluation of surgical intervention must be based on its total effect on the patient. Although there have been immense advances in the surgical options for patients with rheumatoid arthritis over the last several decades, the role of specific procedures in the total picture has many areas of uncertainty and controversy.

Over the years there has been controversy between rheumatologists and surgeons regarding surgery for the correction of rheumatoid problems. There are many reasons for this controversy. This article explores the reasons for the controversy, presents the history of rheumatoid hand surgery, and offers some possible solutions to the problem.

Rheumatoid arthritis (RA) is a progressively destructive disease. Gradual loss of hand function in RA patients affects their ability for self-care and interferes with their productivity in society. The continuing improvement in the medical management of RA has markedly decreased the incidence of RA hand surgery. In contrast to RA, osteoarthritis (OA) has less inflammatory reaction in the joints and is characterized by degradation of cartilage, resulting in joint destruction and osteophyte formation. The initial treatment of OA is medication and therapy. Steroid injection into affected joints can provide short-term relief, though repeat injections carry a cumulative risk of weakening the soft tissue. In this article the authors share their extensive experience in RA and OA hand surgery to provide a clear discussion of the indications and outcomes of its practice.

The elbow is often involved in the progression of rheumatoid arthritis. Because of the elbow's unique role in maneuvering and positioning the hand in space, loss of normal elbow motion, loss of stability, or increased pain with the use of the elbow are all significant sources of impairment in patients with rheumatoid arthritis. The improvements in disease-modifying medications have greatly diminished the prevalence of severe elbow degeneration among patients with rheumatoid arthritis. However, it hasn't been eliminated. In this article the authors discuss strategies for managing it.

Rheumatoid arthritis (RA) may progressively affect all articulations of the wrist. Involvement of the distal radioulnar joint (DRUJ) is common and may be the first clinical signs of symptoms of RA. When the DRUJ is affected by RA, upper extremity function can be affected. Effective surgical management includes the Darrach procedure, the Suave-Kapandji procedure, the hemiresection interposition arthroplasty procedure and extensor tenosynovectomy. The long-term effectiveness of DRUJ arthroplasty is currently unknown.

Wrist involvement in rheumatoid arthritis (RA) is common. Within 2 years of diagnosis, more than half of patients will have wrist pain, and more than 90% will have wrist disease by 10 years. Although wrist involvement is generally thought to be less disabling than RA of the fingers and hand, it can be a significant cause of pain and disability. Severe disease with bony destruction and synovitis in the wrist can also result in soft-tissue problems including tendon ruptures. In addition to musculoskeletal involvement, systemic manifestations of RA can occur. Felty syndrome can result in a low white blood count and splenomegaly in association with RA. New generation, disease-modifying pharmacologic agents offer promise in controlling the disease progression. Surgical treatments for the diseased wrist are aimed at relieving pain and restoring function. Common procedures include: synovectomy and tenosynovectomy, tendon reconstruction, distal ulnar resection and/or distal radioulnar joint reconstruction, partial and full wrist arthrodesis, and total wrist arthroplasty.

Although rheumatoid arthritis causes significant disability for more than 1 million individuals in the United States, prior research regarding surgical treatment options has been limited by study sample size, study design, and methods of comparison. Furthermore, there is wide variation in the referral pattern for hand surgery consideration and type of surgical treatment of rheumatoid hand disease, yet the reasons for these differences are unclear. This review describes the role of outcomes research in rheumatoid hand disease by summarizing variations in surgical treatment, detailing current outcome assessment strategies, and offering potential strategies for designing future studies for rheumatoid hand disease.

Hand Clinics

THE CLINICS ARE NOW AVAILABLE ONLINE!

Access your subscription at:
www.theclinics.com

Preface

Current Concepts in the Treatment of the Rheumatoid Hand, Wrist and Elbow

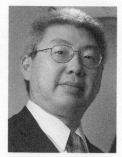

Kevin C. Chung, MD, MS
Guest Editor

The care for the rheumatoid hand has been a fascinating journey for hand surgeons as well as rheumatologists. From a hand surgeon's standpoint, the complexity of the anatomic structures ravaged by rheumatoid arthritis creates an intriguing sequence of deformities that taxes the surgical creativity of hand surgeons to restore function and to ameliorate the continued functional deterioration of the hand and wrist. From a rheumatologist's standpoint, hand conditions are the first sign of the progression of rheumatoid arthritis and effective treatments are available now to slow down—but not to cure—the continual destruction of the hand. For many years, hand surgeons and rheumatologists worked separately to take care of this unique group of patients. Our prior studies have shown that the lack of collaboration between hand surgeons and rheumatologists resulted in uncoordinated and sometimes conflicting care regarding the timing and the outcomes of surgical treatment.

In an effort to bring both specialties closer to gain a consensus regarding the treatment of the rheumatoid hand, this *Hand Clinics* volume is unique because it incorporates the expertise of rheumatologists and hand surgeons by providing their treatment philosophies and sharing rational approaches in addressing common hand and wrist deformities in rheumatoid patients. The authors are all noted authorities in the care of rheumatoid arthritis and they share years of experience to give the most updated information on this topic. Dr David Fox, who is one of the most experienced rheumatologists, gives his perspective on the medical treatment of this condition. The point-counterpoint discussion is provided by Dr Ronald J. Anderson from Brigham and Women's Hospital, who distills his decades of experience from the medical standpoint, whereas Dr Shaw Wilgis shares his surgical perspective from a life-long interest in this disease. Additionally, our colleagues from Europe and rheumatoid hand centers in the United States clarify the treatment approaches for the most complex rheumatoid hand surgery problems.

I am grateful to the publisher of *Hand Clinics*, Debora Dellapena, for seizing the opportunity to publish this unique volume. This volume is not strictly for hand surgeons or strictly for rheumatologists; it is for anyone who has an interest in the care of rheumatoid arthritis and hopes to gain a current perspective on the management of this condition. I also would like to express my personal appreciation to my assistants Pouya Entezami and Phil Clapham, who took on the arduous task in coordinating this particular

Hand Clin 27 (2011) xi–xii
doi:10.1016/j.hcl.2010.10.008

hand.theclinics.com

project. All the contributors of this volume are my personal friends who have dedicated an enormous amount of effort in making this an outstanding product. I have no doubt that you will find this volume enriching and interesting reading to witness the emerging collaboration between rheumatology and hand surgery in treating the rheumatoid hand problem, which will ultimately improve the quality of care for this unique population.

Kevin C. Chung, MD, MS
Section of Plastic Surgery
Department of Surgery
University of Michigan Medical School
2130 Taubman Center
1500 East Medical Center Drive, SPC 5340
Ann Arbor, MI 48109, USA

E-mail address:
kecchung@umich.edu

Historical Perspective on the Etiology of Rheumatoid Arthritis

Pouya Entezami, BS[a], David A. Fox, MD[b],
Philip J. Clapham, BS[a], Kevin C. Chung, MD, MS[c],*

KEYWORDS

- Rheumatoid arthritis • Paintings • Etiology
- Paleopathological

Modern advances in the medical treatment of rheumatoid arthritis (RA) have greatly alleviated patients' symptoms. Development of even more effective remedies could be spurred by the discovery of the etiology of the disease, but the cause of RA remains poorly understood and may involve a combination of genetic, environmental, and stochastic factors. Clues to the etiology of a disease can potentially be obtained from the consideration of its evolution during the development of human civilization. From a historical perspective, evidence for the existence of RA in various eras and locations has come from the analyses of ancient texts, Renaissance artwork, and more recently postmortem remains of hundreds of exhumed skeletons. Unfortunately, much of this research has lacked the rigor of investigative scientific principles, and the findings of this research remain very controversial. Contributions of historical analyses to the development of a cogent etiologic theory of RA have been limited to date.

From this variety of research methodologies, several competing theories concerning the genesis of RA have emerged. One school of thought is that RA is a disease of the modern era and that its pathogenesis is the result of an environmental or a genetic stimulus that did not exist in ancient times. A second theory posits that RA existed among our ancient ancestors but had never been definitively characterized. Most recently, a hybrid theory has developed, which suggests that RA originally developed in indigenous populations in North America and spread to the populations in Europe through the travel of persons and/or goods. The authors have found that most of the literature on the history of RA can be organized into 1 of the 3 categories according to which theory it supports and have named these categories as recent origin, ancient origin, and New World to Old World views.

In this article, the authors analyze this literature with respect to the types and conclusions of the research that has been conducted, present the major points of evidence and conclusions that have been drawn, and trace the evolution of the 3 historical theories of RA. The authors combine a comprehensive overview of paintings and paleopathological investigations (the study of ancient diseases through fossilized remains) with consideration of contemporary immunologic and genetic studies.

Supported in part by a grant from the National Institute of Arthritis and Musculoskeletal and Skin Diseases (R01 AR047328) and a Midcareer Investigator Award in Patient-Oriented Research (K24 AR053120) (K.C.C.).

[a] Section of Plastic Surgery, University of Michigan Health System, 2130 Taubman Center, SPC 5340, 1500 East Medical Center Drive, Ann Arbor, MI 48109-5340, USA
[b] Division of Rheumatology, University of Michigan Medical School, 1500 East Medical Center Drive, Room 3918, Ann Arbor, MI 48109, USA
[c] Section of Plastic Surgery, Department of Surgery, University of Michigan Medical School, 2130 Taubman Center, SPC 5340, 1500 East Medical Center Drive, Ann Arbor, MI 48109-5340, USA
* Corresponding author. Section of Plastic Surgery, Department of Surgery, University of Michigan Medical School, 2130 Taubman Center, SPC 5340, 1500 East Medical Center Drive, Ann Arbor, MI 48109-5340.
E-mail address: kecchung@umich.edu

THE HISTORY OF CLINICAL DESCRIPTIONS OF RA

The first description of RA acknowledged by modern medicine is found in the dissertation of Augustin Jacob Landré-Beauvais[1] in the year 1800. Landré-Beauvais was only 28 years old and a resident physician at the Saltpêtrière asylum in France when he first noticed the symptoms and signs of what we now know to be RA. The investigator examined and treated a handful of patients with severe joint pain that could not be explained by other known maladies at the time (such as rheumatism or osteoarthritis). Unlike gout, this condition mainly affected the poor, affected women more often than men, and had previously been ignored by other physicians who, concerned with earning acclaim and compensation for their work, usually chose to treat more affluent patients.[2] Landré-Beauvais hypothesized that these patients were suffering from a previously uncharacterized condition, which he named *Goutte Asthénique Primitive*, or primary asthenic gout.[1] Although Landré-Beauvais' classification of RA as a relative of gout was inaccurate, his dissertation encouraged other researchers of bone and joint disorders to further study this disease.

The next important contributor to the study of RA was Alfred Garrod,[5] an English physician during the mid- to the late-19th century.[3–5] Alfred Garrod was the first to distinguish gout from other arthritic conditions. He found an excess of uric acid in the blood of patients suffering from gout, but not in the blood of patients with other forms of arthritis.[3,5] In 1859, Alfred Garrod wrote his *Treatise on Nature of Gout and Rheumatic Gout*, wherein he describes these observations. This work differentiated arthritis from gout and also categorized RA as a distinct condition, which he referred to as rheumatic gout. Alfred Garrod's discoveries laid the groundwork for the research on the etiology of RA (rheumatic gout). If this condition could be differentiated from both gout and other forms of arthritis, then a distinct etiology must exist.

Archibald Garrod, the fourth son of Alfred Garrod, also conducted research on RA. In 1890 he authored the extensive *Treatise on Rheumatism and Rheumatoid Arthritis*. In this book the investigator coined the term rheumatoid arthritis to refer to the disease first discovered by Landré-Beauvais and later referred to as rheumatic gout by his father. In the ninety years that had passed since its discovery, more than a dozen terms had been used to describe the same disease. Archibald Garrod chose the term rheumatoid arthritis because it more accurately described the disease's action on the human body. Furthermore, his treatise also delved into the history of RA.[6] Archibald Garrod wrote:

> ...[when some] undifferentiated morbid condition is first described, the characters of which are so striking that it seems well-nigh impossible that they should have been long overlooked it is often suggested that the malady is one of recent development, a new disease which owes its origin to some alteration in the conditions of life...in the case of the disease now to be considered, there is no room for suggestions of this kind, for the evidence of its antiquity is derived, not from mere written descriptions, but from the impress which it has left upon the bones of its victims...

The bones the investigator refers to are ancient skeletal findings from around the world. He discusses bones unearthed in the ruins of Pompeii, skeletons found in a graveyard in Pomerania (near the border of Poland and Germany), bones from ancient Egypt, and even the remains of a Norse Viking found inside his warship, all of which he claimed display skeletal damage indicative of RA.[6] Unfortunately, Archibald Garrod's book only mentions these claims and does not elaborate on the specific supporting evidence. Based on his paleopathological claims, Archibald Garrod proposed that RA was not a disease of the modern era but was present and problematic for our ancestors. His treatise serves as the backbone for the ancient origin school of thought regarding the etiology of RA.

In the twentieth century, the American physician Charles Short challenged Archibald Garrod's paleopathological claims and sought to discredit the ancient origin hypothesis as presented by Archibald Garrod in his *Treatise*. On examination of the original paleontological reports cited in Archibald Garrod's *Treatise*, Short noticed that diagnoses of ankylosing spondylitis (AS), osteoarthritis, and gout had been all confirmed in the skeletal samples. On the other hand, the investigator could not find a definitive diagnosis of RA but rather only claims of RA, which he deemed to be unconvincing. Claiming that Archibald Garrod's ideas were spurious, Short hypothesized that because of the lack of evidence demonstrating otherwise, RA was actually a disease of modern origins.[7] Although other investigators had made similar conjectures in the past, it was Short's work that is most often credited as the basis of the recent origins view of RA. The ancient origins versus recent origins debate persists even today as both sides of the argument continue to develop evidence to support their claims.

EVIDENCE FROM THE LITERATURE AND ART

Although Landré-Beauvais' dissertation is considered to be the first accepted medical report of RA, some researchers have suggested that earlier descriptions are available in ancient texts. The Greek philosopher Hippocrates wrote:

> In the arthritis which generally shows itself about the age of thirty-five there is frequently no great interval between the affection of the hands and feet; both these becoming similar in nature, slender, with little flesh...For the most part their arthritis passeth from the feet to the hands, next the elbows and knees, after these the hip joint. It is incredible how fast the mischief spreads.[3]

It seems possible that Hippocrates was describing a patient with RA. Similar descriptions can be found in the writings of the Greek physician Arataeus, Caesar's physician Scribonius, the Byzantine physician Soranus, Emperor Constantine IX's adviser Michael Psellus, and various other ancient physicians.[3,6,8,9] Many experts consider these texts to be the evidence of RA's existence in ancient times because the writings describe symptoms that closely resemble the signs and symptoms of RA. These researchers believe these ancient writings to be evidence in favor of the ancient origins view of RA etiology. However, opponents claim that these texts offer insufficient support for the prevalence of RA because the vague descriptions do not meet the rigorous scientific standard for making such a claim.[7,10] The role of ancient literature in the etiologic puzzle generally remains anecdotal.

Although archaic, inconsistent terminology makes it difficult to decipher exact diagnoses in premodern writings; artwork may be more successful in displaying a robust demonstration of RA.[11–20] One such painting is *The Three Graces* (1638) by Peter Paul Rubens, which, despite great debate,[21,22] remains as one of the most pronounced pieces of artistic evidence for the existence of RA before Landré-Beauvais' thesis (**Fig. 1**A).[15,23] At a quick glance, the right hand of the left-most "Grace" seems disfigured and poorly represented by the artist. Yet the work of a master painter such as Rubens suggests a different

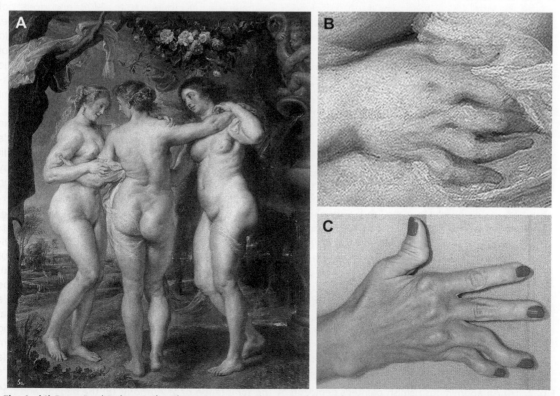

Fig. 1. (A) Peter Paul Rubens' *The Three Graces*, (B) close-up of the left-most figure's hand, and (C) a patient with similar pattern of RA damage as in the picture.

reason. Exploring Rubens' history as an artist reveals that he usually adhered to realism and depicted his models in a realistic way. From an anatomic perspective, the fingers are positioned in an unnatural way. The fingers on the right hand are both flexed and in hyperextension (see **Fig. 1**B). Although this finger position is possible if a digit has suffered some injury, an injury of every finger is unlikely. This observation makes a diagnosis of RA much more believable. **Fig. 1**C shows a patient with RA with a hand deformity similar to that seen in the hand of the woman in Rubens' painting. It is possible that the model Rubens used for this painting suffered from RA.

The most convincing case of RA during the Renaissance is a depiction of *The Temptation of St. Anthony* by an anonymous painter (mid-15th to early 16th century) from the Flemish-Dutch School, as reported by Drs Dequeker and Rico in 1992 (**Fig. 2**A).[12] The beggar in the left-hand corner is the subject in question (see **Fig. 2**B). Particularly striking is the deformity of the beggar's right hand, showing wrist luxation, ulnar deviation, and finger contractures (see **Fig. 2**C). This pattern is very similar to that seen in many patients with RA (see **Fig. 2**D, E). **Table 1** lists paintings by other artists who experts have claimed to show signs of RA-induced deformities.

Conclusions derived from paintings must be considered carefully because art pieces are not necessarily scientifically sound evidence. It is important to remember that what an artist depicts in his or her work reflects personal stylistic choices.[12] Artists do not always set out to document their surroundings. Rather they may be more focused on creating dramatic, expressive, and beautiful results. Inferences made from paintings are typically met by critics who have, often correctly, shown that some physical features depicted in paintings are purely artistic convention and hold no medical importance.[10,24,25]

Furthermore, some researchers attribute the conditions portrayed in these paintings as evidence of other rheumatic diseases (such as rheumatic fever or gout) and not necessarily RA. Although these diseases may manifest themselves similarly to RA, their onsets, pathologies, and treatments are very distinct. For example, rheumatic fever generally affects young children and is caused by a streptococcal infection, yet its physical manifestations may resemble RA in certain patients. Because of these complexities, it is generally difficult to affirm an artistic depiction of a medical condition as being RA from paintings. Moreover, the deformities depicted by Rubens and others do not correspond to the most severe

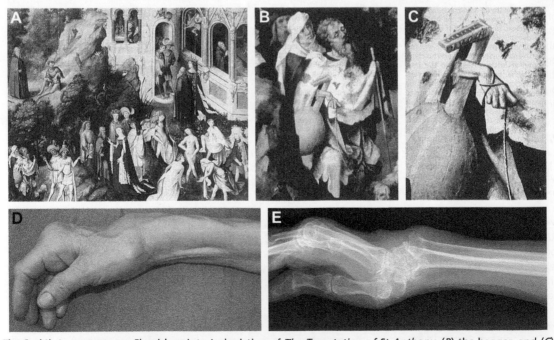

Fig. 2. (*A*) An anonymous Flemish painter's depiction of *The Temptation of St Anthony*, (*B*) the beggar, and (*C*) close-up of the beggar's deformed hand showing slight ulnar deviation, finger contractures, and wrist luxation. (*D, E*) Patient with a similar pattern of RA damage as in the picture.

Table 1
Paintings that include human figures with characteristics suggested of being caused by RA

Artist	Title	Year Painted
Anonymous	*The Temptation of St Anthony*	15th—16th century CE
Guiseppe Maria Crespi	*The Holy Family*	17th—18th century CE
Jacob Jordaens	*The Painter's Family*	1620
Cornelisz Moeyaert	*Portrait of Siebrandus Sixtius*	1631
Rembrandt Harmenszoon van Rijn	*Portrait of Maria Brockenolle*	1634
Peter Paul Rubens	*Rubens' final self-portrait*	17th century CE
Peter Paul Rubens	*The Three Graces*	1638

Data from Refs.[12–16,19,59]

and mutilating deformities that RA can produce. If RA existed in Rubens' milieu, one might expect that its most severe and spectacular changes would have attracted the attention of artists.

Nevertheless, visual arts have been used in previous etiologic research for various other medical conditions.[14,23,25] For example, the figures from Michelangelo di Lodovico Buonarroti Simoni's (1475–1564) paintings on the ceiling of the Sistine Chapel show signs of goiter, which endocrinologists have used as evidence pertinent to the historical epidemiology of thyroid disease.[23] Paintings analyzed by both medical experts and art historians can offer reliable information that other methods of research may not be able to provide. In the case of RA, paintings may suggest the presence of the disease in ancient times and are cited by some experts in support of the ancient origin view of the disease. However, a definitive diagnosis of RA is impossible from these paintings because of the similarities between the presentation of RA and that of other rheumatic diseases.

PALEOPATHOLOGICAL EVIDENCE

In addition to the analyses of historical medical writings and paintings, postmortem investigations provide a venue for gathering scientific data about a disease's historical prevalence. The lack of widely accepted ancient medical texts regarding RA has forced researchers to turn to paleopathological studies. Due to the nature of buried skeletal remains, which generally lack soft tissues, bone and joint diseases (including RA) are typically easy to study on post-mortem specimens.

Two preliminary paleopathological studies independently performed by Professor Flinders Petrie and Sir Armand Ruffer in the late-19th and early-20th centuries discuss human remains from Egypt that demonstrate skeletal damage similar to that

of RA.[26–31] Ruffer was given skeletal samples from 7 different burial sites in Egypt, which included Egyptian, Greek, and Macedonian remains. On examination of the skeletons, the investigator noticed severe lesions and eburnation of the joints, which he concluded were suggestive of RA. A similar approach was used for the discoveries by Professor Petrie and comparable results were found. Unfortunately, these pioneering studies were done before the development of modern paleopathological methods. Furthermore, it was not until the 1970s that RA and AS were conclusively differentiated through genetic studies.[32] Close inspection of Ruffer's work reveals many potential cases of AS but not one definitive case of RA. Ruffer and Petrie's works are generally not considered to be convincing evidence for RA in ancient times. However, their work demonstrated that evidence of rheumatic diseases could be identified in ancient human remains.

Since the work of Ruffer and Petrie, more than a dozen paleopathological studies of RA have been conducted. These recent studies have used better-defined criteria for establishing RA in archeological samples to counter the criticisms of the preliminary studies. In the earlier studies, researchers had compared what they saw in paleontological samples (which had endured the elements for centuries) with damage they had seen in fresh cadavers, which meant that a diagnosis was being made without considering the condition or preservation of the skeleton. This diagnosis proved problematic because some signs of RA described in these first studies could be attributed to postmortem erosion, a concern that led to the discrediting of many of the early studies. During the mid-20th century, researchers began using radiography as the common method of comparing skeletal remains with living patients. However, this comparison also entailed that their observations were dependent on the nature of soft tissue found in a living patient (ie, the effect of soft tissue on radiographs used for radiological imaging).[33,34] Thus, it was proposed that the signs indicative of RA damage seen on dry skeletons may not have been caused by RA. These methods and criteria have changed significantly over the last few decades. Prerequisites proposed for diagnosing RA in skeletons include the presence of the following features (expanded from the list developed by Arcini in 1992)[35–39]:

1. Subchondral cysts
2. Erosions/periarticular sinuses in affected joints
3. Rebuilding and/or presence of osteophytes
4. Severe periarticular bone fragmentation or sinuses
5. Ulnar deviation of the metacarpophalangeal joints
6. Traces in cartilage-supporting bone tissues of a multiarticular joint as evidence of the disease's effect on all the articular facets of the joint (distinguishing it from osteoarthritis)
7. Osseous ankylosis of joints (especially carpal and metacarpal)
8. Eburnation
9. Multiple joints that are bilaterally affected.

This list is a compilation of the most used criteria for diagnosing RA in paleopathological studies. However, subchondral cysts, eburnation, and ankylosis are seen in other forms of arthritis, such as osteoarthritis and AS, whereas osteophytes are rarely seen in RA but are typical of osteoarthritis. Thus, this list of radiographic abnormalities lacks specificity for RA. Most samples judged to suggest RA display only a few of these criteria, which some researchers nonetheless deem to be sufficient evidence for making a diagnosis of RA.

Notwithstanding these limitations, a few reports of RA in ancient remains hold up under scrutiny. The most striking case of RA found in paleopathological samples was described by Arcini in 1992.[36] **Fig. 3** shows the right hand from a skeleton found in Europe, displaying both ulnar deviation and damage of the index finger. This pattern of damage makes these remains the most likely case of RA found in Europe before Landré-Beauvais' description.

One deficiency of paleontological studies is that the samples are not always ideally preserved and it is difficult to construct complete skeletal sets. Given that RA most prominently affects the hands and feet, which are usually difficult to find, skeletons with the potential to show signs of RA are particularly hard to come by.[40] Another perplexing issue for paleontological researchers is distinguishing RA from other erosive arthropathies. Similar to

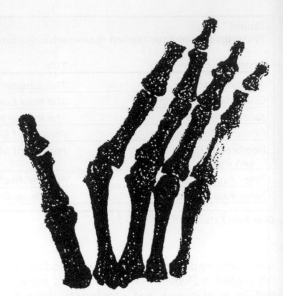

Fig. 3. Right hand of skeleton showing ulnar deviation and damage of the second finger, which are indicative of RA. (*From* Arcini C. Rheumatoid arthritis—rare findings from Scanian skeletal remains from Viking and medieval times. Sydsvenska Medicinhist Sallsk Arsskr 1992;18:11–21; with permission.)

the problems that arise when considering artistic representations, other diseases sometimes result in a similar pattern of skeletal damage. Hence, disease-specific diagnoses must be justified by the level of detail preserved in the remains.[29,37,41] Some critics disagree with the results of these studies because of disparities in the methods used to infer RA in skeletal samples.[41–43] Still others object based on their own research having found no indications of RA.[44]

Nonetheless, the development of rigorous scientific techniques within paleopathology (a specialty field within medical anthropology) has uncovered samples from around the world that demonstrate skeletal damage that may be suggestive of RA. By taking into consideration the expertise of anthropologists, physicians can distinguish skeletal damage caused by diseases from that caused by the elements. This distinguishability has greatly increased the validity of more recent studies. **Table 2** includes a comprehensive list of all paleopathological studies that claim the presence of skeletal damage indicative of RA. Reviewing the figures and text from each study reveals that many of the cases listed in **Table 2** are ambiguous and generally not specific for RA. Still, there are some convincing cases from around the world that demonstrate signs of RA preceding Landré-Beauvais' description of RA by several hundred years, thereby favoring the ancient origin view of RA etiology.[45]

Table 2
Published paleopathological studies of RA

Date of Samples	Year Published	Location	Hypothesis Supported
4000–1000 BCE	1917	Egypt	Ancient origin
3000–1000 BCE	1988	Alabama	New World to Old World
2750–2625 BCE	1897	Egypt	Ancient origin
2500–1900 BCE	1988	Sweden	Ancient origin
2290–2040 BCE	1990	Kentucky	New World to Old World
1300 BCE	1940	Lower Egypt	Ancient origin
800 BCE	1988	Ohio	New World to Old World
400–1 BCE	1985	Denmark	Ancient origin
339–210 BCE	1979	Sicily	Ancient origin
100 BCE	1983	England	Ancient origin
700–1450 CE	1989	Sudan	Ancient origin
900–1536 CE	1992	Denmark/Sweden	Ancient origin
1400 CE	1981	England	Ancient origin
1500 CE	2002	Italy	Ancient origin
1666 CE	2009	Italy	Ancient origin

Data from Refs.[28,30,35,36,38–40,48,49,60–65]

Different interpretations of the findings in **Table 2** by various experts have led to the development of a third school of thought regarding the etiology of RA, the New World to Old World transfer concept.[46,47] Proponents of this view argue that because some of the oldest paleopathological specimens displaying RA were found in the Americas, RA must have been transmitted to the Old World through an unspecified vector after initial discovery of the Americas by Columbus.[38,48,49] However, studies that have found the presence of RA in the Old World before Columbus' voyage in 1492 may potentially discredit this theory. Undeterred, the New World to Old World idea has recently gained momentum, especially since contact between the New World and the Old World certainly preceded the voyages of Columbus by several centuries.

CONTEMPORARY RESEARCH

Recent research on the origins and etiology of RA has begun to approach the issue from a molecular perspective.[41,50] It has long been hypothesized that some genetic component plays a role in the onset of RA. For example, it has been known since the first descriptions of RA that women are more likely to be affected than men by a ratio of 3:1.[1,27,40] Research over the past 35 years has shown an association between RA and a group of major histocompatibility complex (MHC class II) cell surface receptors encoded by alleles of the HLA-DR locus on chromosome 6.[41,51–53] The MHC locus is highly polymorphic, and different populations differ in allele frequency. The particular set of alleles that individuals carry is highly predictive of their potential to develop RA, and susceptibility alleles are found in individuals within every population. Although many other genes contribute to RA susceptibility, the most important contribution comes from the MHC locus.

Other studies have shown that genetics is not the sole determinant of RA.[50,53] Microbial pathogens, including bacteria, as well as various viruses (retroviruses, parvovirus B19, rubella, Epstein-Barr, and other herpesviruses) have been implicated as potential triggers of RA.[50,52–55] The mechanism of action of these events is still unclear, and it is plausible that infections are not causative and, rather, patients with RA may just be more prone to infections. Thus, the suggested pathogens have only been circumstantially implicated as playing a triggering role. Hypotheses that correlate the onset of RA to an infections trigger will remain speculative until a discrete pathogen has been found. Determining what, if any, role bacterial and viral infections play in the onset of RA is still a developing area of research.

Smoking has been implicated as another potential environmental trigger. In particular, smoking has been linked to the incidence of RA in individuals with the HLA susceptibility allele, termed the shared epitope (SE).[56] In the context of this discussion, the influence of smoking on RA heavily favors the New World to Old World view because smoking was introduced to Europe only after Columbus' discovery of the Americas. However, this correlation is not perfect because about one-third of the patients with RA do not have the HLA-DR SE gene. Also, not all people with RA smoke, although effects of second-hand smoke or similar environmental toxins could potentially be important in nonsmoker subjects with RA. Thus, smoking may not necessarily be a uniform cause of RA, but instead one of the several environmental triggers involved in the genesis of RA. A possible mechanism for the effect of smoking in RA may be through induction of the formation of citrullinated autoantigens, the most specific target of immune autoreactivity yet identified in RA. As it stands, this concept is still under development. To develop a more definitive conclusion, stronger evidence is needed to flesh out an immunopathogenic pathway that connects smoking, RA, and autoimmune responses.

It has been suggested that the aforementioned causes (smoking, infectious triggers) are not actually causes but rather risk factors.[50] This suggestion implies that RA could have been present in the populations of both the ancient New and Old Worlds, albeit very rare in the Old World in the absence of important environmental triggers. After the opening of trade routes between the hemispheres, certain risk factors (especially tobacco) could have been introduced to Europe, which contributed to the eventual appearance of RA as a more common disease in the Old World. This model is attractive and is consistent with current hypotheses regarding the etiology of RA. However, as with the other suggested models, this model must be explored much further.

CURRENT HYPOTHESIS

RA generally begins to manifest in individuals between the ages of 30 and 65 years.[57] The estimated average life expectancy was just lesser than 30 years when RA was first described in the year 1800.[58] Therefore, it is possible that individuals who would have developed RA in ancient times died before the onset of the disease. This observation could partly explain why RA may have been much less common in previous centuries. Combined with the aforementioned paleopathological evidence showing the prevalence of RA in antiquity, a reasonable conclusion seems to be that RA was problematic for our ancestors in ancient times but likely for very few of them.

The unresolved question is about the generation of ancestors included. The New World to Old

World concept proposes that an infectious trigger was transferred from the New World to Europe via trade goods (eg, smoking tobacco), contaminated supplies, or travelers who picked up RA-inducing bacteria or viruses. Despite the plausibility of many of these arguments, discoveries of skeletons demonstrating RA in the Old World before the discovery of the Americas suggest that these transferred environmental (and perhaps also genetic) factors were not absolute prerequisites for the development of RA.

By combining the conclusions from paleopathological studies with those from advanced immunologic and genetic analyses, a modified and updated version of the ancient origin view now stands as the best-supported theory concerning the historical epidemiology of RA. The current hypothesis consists of the following principles:

1. RA is not a disease of recent origin and was both present and problematic hundreds, possibly thousands, of years ago, potentially with a geographic distribution distinct from its current profile.
2. RA occurs as a response to an environmental stimulus or stimuli experienced by genetically susceptible individuals.
3. The identities and origins of these stimuli or inciting events are still incompletely known, although tantalizing clues have emerged.
4. Distinct environmental triggers may be important in subsets of patients with RA. For example, smoking may be a more important risk factor in patients with RA who carry an MHC allele that encodes the SE and who have autoantibodies to citrulline-containing proteins. Thus, the historical analysis of RA needs to incorporate the likely possibility that what is currently defined as RA is more than one disease.

This framework allows research to be directed toward a more expanded set of possible etiologic causes that may have been overlooked if one adheres strictly to any of the 3 previously held hypotheses concerning the history of RA. Potentially, an integration of molecular insights and historical epidemiology may provide new clues for identifying the etiology of RA.

REFERENCES

1. Landré-Beauvais AJ. The first description of rheumatoid arthritis. Unabridged text of the doctoral dissertation presented in 1800. Joint Bone Spine 2001;68:130–42.
2. Kahn MF A. J. Landré-Beauvais. Joint Bone Spine 2001;68:143.

3. Copeman WS. A short history of gout. Berkeley (Los Angeles): University of California Press; 1964.
4. Storey GD. Alfred Baring Garrod (1819–1907). Rheumatology 2001;40:1189–90.
5. Garrod AB. Treatise on nature of gout and rheumatic gout. London: Walton and Maberly; 1859.
6. Garrod AE. A treatise on rheumatism and rheumatoid arthritis. London: Charles Griffin and Company; 1890.
7. Short CL. The antiquity of rheumatoid arthritis. Arthritis Rheum 1974;17(3):193–205.
8. Caughey DE. The arthritis of Constantine IX. Ann Rheum Dis 1974;33:77–80.
9. Soranus of Ephesus. On acute diseases and on chronic diseases, translated into Latin by Caelius Aurelianus (fifth century AD). English translation by IE Drabkin. Chicago: University of Chicago Press; 1950.
10. Snorrason E. Landre Beauvais and his "Goutte Asthenique Primitive". Acta Med Scand 1952; 142(Suppl 256):115–8.
11. Alarcón-Segovia D, Laffón A, Alcocer-Varela J. Probable depiction of juvenile arthritis by Sandro Botticelli. Arthritis Rheum 1983;26(10):1266–8.
12. Dequeker J, Rico H. Rheumatoid arthritis–like deformities in an early 16th-century painting of the Flemish-Dutch school. JAMA 1992;268(2):249–51.
13. Hayakawa S, Komine-Aizawa S, Osaka S, et al. Rembrandt's Maria Bockenolle has a butterfly rash and digital deformities: overlapping syndrome of rheumatoid arthritis and systemic lupus erythematosus. Med Hypotheses 2007;68:906–9.
14. Dequeker J. Medicine and the artist. Age Ageing 2008;37:4–5.
15. Appelboom T. Hypothesis: Rubens—one of the first victims of an epidemic of rheumatoid arthritis that started in the 16th-17th century? Rheumatology 2004;44:681–3.
16. Rubinstein HM, Blair SJ. The hand in art. J Hand Surg Am 1985;10A(4):589.
17. Levine H. Art, artists, and arthritis. Md Med 2002; 3(2):40.
18. Levine H. Art, artists, and arthritis. Md Med 2002; 3(3):45.
19. Rubens. The artist and arthritis. Sci News 1981; 119(8):117.
20. Boonen A, Rest J, Dequeker J, et al. How Renoir coped with rheumatoid arthritis. Br Med J 1997; 315:1704–8.
21. Appelboom T. Style versus substance in artistic depiction: reply. Rheumatology 2005;44(11):1465.
22. Rothschild B. Style versus substance in artistic depiction. Rheumatology 2005;44(11):1464.
23. Slater V, Ramachandran M. Medical conditions in works of art. Br Med J 2008;315:1704–8.
24. Leden I. Doubts about Sandro Boticelli's depiction of juvenile rheumatoid arthritis. Arthritis Rheum 1984; 27(10):1197–8.
25. Weisman M, P RJ, Steinberg L, et al. International symposium: art, history, and antiquity of rheumatic diseases. Clin Rheumatol 1986;5:278–94.
26. Bridges PS. Prehistoric arthritis in the Americas. Ann Rev Anthropol 1922;21:67–91.
27. Barr J. An address on rheumatoid arthritis. Br Med J 1913;1(2728):733–5.
28. Ruffer A. Arthritis deformans and spondylitis in ancient Egypt. J Pathol 1918;22:152–96.
29. Karsh RS, McCarthy JD. Archaeology and arthritis. Arch Intern Med 1960;105:640–4.
30. May WP. Rheumatoid arthritis (osteitis deformans) affecting bones 5500 years old. Br Med J 1897; 2(1927):1631–2.
31. Domen RE. Paleopathological evidence of rheumatoid arthritis. JAMA 1981;246(17):1899.
32. Schlosstein L, Terasaki PI, Bluestone R, et al. High association of an HL-A antigen, W27, with ankylosing spondylitis. N Engl J Med 1973;288:704–6.
33. Ortner DJ, Utermohle CJ. Polyarticular inflammatory arthritis in a pre-Columbian skeleton from Kodiak Island, Alaska, U.S.A. Am J Phys Anthropol 1981; 56:23–31.
34. Rothschild BM. Paleopathology, its character and contribution to understanding and distinguishing among rheumatologic diseases: perspectives on rheumatoid arthritis and spondyloarthropathy. Clin Exp Rheumatol 1995;13:652–62.
35. Thould AK, Thould BT. Arthritis in Roman Britain. Br Med J 1983;287:24–31.
36. Arcini C. Rheumatoid arthritis—rare findings from Scanian skeletal remains from Viking and medieval times. Sydsven Medicinhist Sallsk Arsskr 1992;18: 11–21.
37. Lagier R. Bone eburnation in rheumatic diseases: a guiding trace in today's radiological diagnosis and in paleopathology. Clin Rheumatol 2006;25: 127–31.
38. Rothschild BM, Woods RJ. Symmetrical erosive disease in archaic Indians: the origin of rheumatoid arthritis in the New World. Semin Arthritis Rheum 1990;19(5):278–84.
39. Giuffra V, Vitiello A, Giusiani S, et al. Rheumatoid arthritis, Klippel-Feil syndrome and Pott's disease in Cardinal Carlo de' Medici (1595–1666). Clin Exp Rheumatol 2009;27:594–602.
40. Bennike P. Paleopathology of Danish skeletons: a comparative study of demography, disease, and injury. Copenhagen (Denmark): Akademisk Forlag; 1985.
41. Ortner DJ, Tuross N, Stix AI. New approaches to the study of disease in archeological New World populations. Hum Biol 1992;64(3):337–60.
42. Duncan H. Letter to the editor. Paleopathol Newsl 1979;25:10–1.
43. Klepinger L. Letter to the editor. Paleopathol Newsl 1979;26:6–7.

44. Rothschild BM, Arriaza B, Woods RJ, et al. Spondyloarthropathy identified as the etiology of Nubian erosive arthropathies. Am J Phys Anthropol 1999; 109:259–67.

45. Rogers J, Dieppe P. Skeletal palaeopathology and the rheumatic diseases: where are we now? Ann Rheum Dis 1990;49:885–6.

46. Kramar C, Lagier R, Baud CA. Rheumatic diseases in neolithic and medieval populations of Western Switzerland. Zeitschrift fur Rheumatologie 1990;49: 338–45.

47. Domen RE. The antiquity and origins of rheumatoid arthritis. JAMA 1992;268(19):2649.

48. Rothschild BM, Turner KR, DeLuca MA. Symmetrical erosive polyarthritis in the late archaic period of Alabama. Science 1988;241:1498–501.

49. Woods RJ, Rothschild BM. Population analysis of symmetrical erosive arthritis in Ohio Woodland Indians (1200 years ago). J Rheumatol 1988;15(8): 1258–63.

50. Fox DA. Etiology and pathogenesis of rheumatoid arthritis. In: Koopman WJ, editor. Arthritis and allied conditions: a textbook of rheumatology, vol. 1. 15th edition. Philadelphia: Lippincott Williams & Wilkins; 2005. p. 1089–107.

51. Reveille JD. The genetic contribution to the pathogenesis of rheumatoid arthritis. Curr Opin Rheumatol 1998;10:187–200.

52. Condemi JJ. The autoimmune diseases. JAMA 1992;268(20):2882–92.

53. Moreland LW. Rheumatoid arthritis: epidemiology, pathogenesis, and treatment. London: ReMEDICA Publishing; 2001.

54. Álvarez-Lafuente R, Fernández-Gutiérrez B, Miguel S, et al. Potential relationship between herpes viruses and rheumatoid arthritis: analysis with a quantitative real time polymerase chain reaction. Ann Rheum Dis 2005;64:1357–9.

55. Balandraud N, Roudier J, Roudier C. Epstein-Barr virus and rheumatoid arthritis. Autoimmun Rev 2004;3:362–7.

56. Klareskog L, Stolt P, Lundberg K, et al. A new model for an etiology for rheumatoid arthritis: smoking may trigger HLA-DR (shared epitope) restricted immune reactions to autoantigens modified by citrullination. Arthritis Rheum 2006;54(1):38–46.

57. Majithia V, Geraci SA. Rheumatoid arthritis: diagnosis and management. Am J Med 2007;120:936–9.

58. Riley JC. Estimates of regional and global life expectancy. Popul Dev Rev 2005;31(3):537–43.

59. Dequeker J. Siebrandus Sixtius: evidence of rheumatoid arthritis of the robust reaction type in a seventeenth century Dutch priest. Ann Rheum Dis 1991; 51:561–2.

60. Hormell RS. Notes on the history of rheumatism and gout. N Engl J Med 1940;223(19):754–60.

61. Klepinger LL. Paleopathologic evidence for the evolution of rheumatoid arthritis. Am J Phys Anthropol 1979;50:119–22.

62. Rogers J, Watt I, Dieppe P. Arthritis in Saxon and mediaeval skeletons. Br Med J 1981;283:19–26.

63. Leden I, Persson E, Persson O. Aspects of the history of rheumatoid arthritis in the light of recent osteo-archeological finds. Scand J Rheumatol 1988;17:341–52.

64. Kilgore L. Possible case of rheumatoid arthritis from Sudanese Nubia. Am J Phys Anthropol 1989;79: 177–83.

65. Ciranni R, Garbini F, Neri E, et al. The "Braids Lady" of Arezzo: a case of rheumatoid arthritis in a 16th century mummy. Clin Exp Rheumatol 2002;20: 745–52.

Advances in the Medical Treatment of Rheumatoid Arthritis

J. Michelle Kahlenberg, MD, PhD, David A. Fox, MD*

KEYWORDS

- Rheumatoid arthritis
- Disease-modifying antirheumatic drugs
- Biologic therapy • Perioperative management

Rheumatoid arthritis (RA) is an inflammatory arthritis that affects nearly 1% of the world's adults. RA is characterized by symmetric polyarticular inflammation of the synovium, typically of the small joints of the hands (metacarpophalangeal [MCP] and proximal interphalangeal [PIP]), wrists, and feet. This inflammation results in pain and stiffness, and can lead to progressive joint damage resulting in deformities and loss of function. Associated organ damage also contributes to severe disability. In addition, chronic inflammation secondary to RA can lead to an increased risk of cardiovascular disease and changes in bone metabolism.

Over the past 2 decades, the treatment of RA has been revolutionized by advances in the understanding of its pathologic mechanisms and the development of drugs that target them. These newer medications have shown great promise at improving disease outcomes, but they come with notable side effects that can pose long-term treatment challenges and difficulties in the perioperative arena. In this article, the major manifestations of RA and the current medical options for management are discussed. Complications from treatment are then reviewed and special consideration is given to perioperative medication recommendations.

ARTICULAR AND SYSTEMIC EFFECTS OF RA
Articular Manifestations

Inflammation and subsequent destruction of synovial joints is the hallmark of RA. Why the immune system is lured to attack and destroy still remains unknown, but great strides have been made in understanding the pathogenesis of this disease. Inflammation of the synovial tissue involves interactions between macrophages, T and B lymphocytes, synovial fibroblasts, and other cells of the inflamed synovium such as mast cells, dendritic cells, and plasma cells. Neutrophils are rare in RA synovial tissue but abundant in RA synovial fluid. These cell-cell interactions occur both through direct cell-cell contact, as well as through the effects of secreted mediators. Proinflammatory cytokines, such as tumor necrosis factor-α (TNFα), interleukin (IL)-1, and IL-6, orchestrate synovial inflammation and stimulate cartilage degradation. This process occurs through formation of a distinct tissue termed synovial pannus that invades cartilage with the assistance of proteolytic enzymes. Concurrently osteoclasts, which can form within the pannus through fusion of monocytic precursors, invade bone and cause periarticular erosions.

Supported by grants from the Arthritis Foundation and from the NIH (NIAMS AR38477).
The authors have no conflicts of interest to disclose.
Division of Rheumatology, University of Michigan, 3918 Taubman Center, 1500 East Medical Center, SPC 5358, Ann Arbor, MI 48109-5358, USA
* Corresponding author.
E-mail address: dfox@umich.edu

Hand Clin 27 (2011) 11–20
doi:10.1016/j.hcl.2010.09.002
0749-0712/11/$ — see front matter

RA can involve most synovial joints, but rarely the distal interphalangeal joints or the thoracic, lumbar, and sacral spine. The most commonly affected joints include the MCP and PIP joints of the hands and wrists, and metatarsophalangeal joints of the feet. Joint destruction begins early in the disease, with erosive changes often seen after only 6 months. The clinical examination can disclose synovial thickening and swelling, indicators of joint inflammation. At the time of presentation, nearly 70% of radiographs can be normal, but magnetic resonance imaging (MRI) and ultrasonography with power Doppler have higher sensitivity in detecting smaller erosions and synovial inflammation, and may reveal changes even when radiographs are normal.[1] If RA is left untreated, progression to joint destruction, subluxation, and severe disability are the likely outcomes.

Inflammation of tendon sheaths also contributes to RA pathology. Tenosynovitis of the flexor tendons can lead to trigger finger, and weakening of the extensor tendons of the hands from chronic inflammation can lead to tendon ruptures. Damage to supporting structures of the joints and tendons of the hand contribute to the formation of boutonniere and swan-neck deformities. Carpal tunnel syndrome secondary to median nerve compression by surrounding inflammation is also a common complication in RA patients.

Bone Manifestations

The bones of RA patients are affected in both a local and systemic manner. At a local level, factors that stimulate osteoclasts causing increased bone resorption are released from inflammatory and fibroblastic pannus cells.[2] In addition, inflammatory cytokines prevent a compensatory increase in the rate of periarticular bone formation, resulting in net bone loss. This inhibition of osteoblastic activity occurs through a combination of impaired mineralization and impaired osteoblast differentiation.[3] These processes combine to result in both periarticular osteopenia, one of the first radiographic signs of RA, and periarticular erosions, the hallmark of RA joint destruction.[1] The use of disease-modifying agents to induce clinical remission allows for restoration of normal function of osteoclasts and osteoblasts, and may result in repair of erosive damage.[4]

Bony changes in RA patients are not only seen in a periarticular distribution. RA is a known risk factor for osteoporosis, with up to 30% of patients affected by some estimates.[5] Most studies agree that, unlike postmenopausal osteoporosis, the risk of osteoporosis in RA patients is greater at the femoral neck than in the spine, but both areas can be involved. Disease duration and severity, sex, body mass, and the use of corticosteroids all influence the risk of osteoporosis in RA patients.[5,6]

An additional consideration is that many RA patients are on bisphosphonate therapy for osteoporosis or prevention of glucocorticoid-mediated bone loss. Research into the impact of bisphosphonate use in patients undergoing surgical procedures is ongoing. Osteonecrosis of the jaw in patients on bisphosphonates undergoing dental surgery has been a specific concern, but the consequences of manipulation of the peripheral skeleton in patients on these medications are still incompletely understood. Most research into this topic is in animal systems, and there are suggestions that although bone healing is not prevented, there are differences in bone quality after bisphosphonate exposure.[7]

Airway Manifestations

The presence of airway disease in RA is estimated to affect 20% to 30% of patients. Manifestations can include cricoarytenoid arthritis, pulmonary fibrosis, and small airway disease, typically seen as bronchiolitis obliterans on histopathology, and obstructive abnormalities on lung function testing.[8,9] Lung disease is more frequent in RA patients who are male, seropositive, smoke, and have long-standing disease.[9] Some types of RA-associated lung disease are steroid responsive, but some patients have a progressive course leading to end-stage fibrosis and death.[10] In addition to lung disease secondary to RA, patients are also at risk for pulmonary toxicities from RA-related medications, including methotrexate, leflunomide, and even anti-TNF medications.[9]

Cardiovascular Manifestations

RA patients have a 40% increased risk of mortality as compared with the general population after 20 years of disease. This increased risk of mortality is primarily attributed to an increased incidence of cardiovascular disease.[11] A recent cohort study has suggested that the risk of cardiovascular events in RA patients is twofold higher than the general population, equivalent to the risk of patients with diabetes.[12] The propensity for vascular changes is found even in newly diagnosed patients, indicating that common mechanisms may exist, linking synovitis resulting in joint destruction with endothelial dysfunction resulting in atherosclerosis.[13]

The risk of cardiovascular disease and death increases with more severe disease and elevated inflammatory markers.[11,14] Despite improved treatments for the symptoms of RA, the mortality risk has not improved over the past 2 decades. Whether this continued risk of death reflects an inability to control cardiovascular risk factors with immunomodulatory treatment or a lack of long-term follow-up in patients treated with newer medications remains to be determined. In addition, the optimal management of traditional cardiovascular risk factors, such as elevated cholesterol, has not been determined for RA patients.

PHARMACEUTICAL OPTIONS FOR THE TREATMENT OF RA
Disease-Modifying Antirheumatic Drugs

Disease-modifying antirheumatic drugs (DMARDs) became the mainstay of RA treatment in the 1970s. As a group, they have been shown to decrease inflammation and slow radiographic progression, but the degree to which this is accomplished is variable. The timing of DMARD initiation has been debated, but current consensus suggests that the earlier the treatment can be initiated, the better the overall outcome for clinical improvement and prevention of erosive disease.[15] The initial 15 months of RA are critical for initiation and escalation of DMARD therapy in order to achieve acceptable long-term outcomes.[16] A major difficulty in treating patients with RA is that it is currently impossible to predict which patients will respond to which medication regimen. Current research is ongoing to develop patient-specific disease signatures via genetic and proteomic approaches; however, the practical application of such advances has not been achieved. Thus, practice guidelines typically recommend starting with conventional DMARD treatment before addition or substitution of biologic DMARD medications. Of importance, the use of DMARDs in combination rather than monotherapy is more effective in achieving improved clinical outcomes as well as slowing radiographic progression.[17] Conventional DMARDs can be combined with each other and/or with biologic DMARDs. Each DMARD has its own unique toxicities and required monitoring, which is summarized in **Table 1**.

The mainstay of DMARD therapy is methotrexate, which is administered weekly, either orally or subcutaneously. Its use began for RA in the 1970s, and it has shown sustained benefits for at least 50% of RA patients who receive it. Known as an antagonist of folic acid metabolism, its effects in inflammatory diseases may actually be secondary to the induction of adenosine release and the inhibition of polyamines.[18] Typically it is well tolerated and most gastrointestinal side effects can be mitigated by subcutaneous administration if needed. Folic acid is coadministered to avoid toxicities secondary to inhibition of rapid cell turnover. Monitoring for liver toxicity is advised, but unless a patient has other risk factors for liver damage (hepatitis B or C infection, alcohol consumption), serious liver damage from methotrexate is rare. The use of methotrexate has been shown to slow radiographic progression and improve clinical outcomes of RA patients. DMARD monotherapy with methotrexate is sufficient for about one-third of RA patients; however, as mentioned elsewhere in this article, its effect is more pronounced when used either in combination therapy with other DMARDs or in conjunction with a biologic agent.[17,19,20]

Leflunomide is a DMARD that acts specifically on lymphocytes by blocking pyrimidine synthesis. As a monotherapy, it generates similar improvements in clinical measures and radiographic scores to methotrexate.[20,21] Often, it is used in place of methotrexate in combination with other DMARDs or biologic DMARDs when side effects of methotrexate limit its use. As with methotrexate, preexisting liver disease, alcohol abuse, pregnancy (or inadequate contraception), or active infection are contraindications to the use of leflunomide. Unlike methotrexate, leflunomide may be used in patients with mild to moderate renal insufficiency. A unique property of leflunomide is its prolonged half-life secondary to binding of plasma proteins and enterohepatic circulation. Thus, an elimination protocol using cholestyramine is often needed when circumstances warrant rapid drug elimination such as during serious infections or pregnancy.

Hydroxychloroquine (HCQ) is a mild DMARD that is well tolerated and has minimal side effects. HCQ has been shown to be effective in improving joint pain and function, but has not been shown to slow radiographic damage.[20] Thus, the use of HCQ is recommended in conjunction with other DMARDs or for very mild RA that does not demonstrate ongoing joint damage. HCQ may protect RA patients from the subsequent development of diabetes, and it has been noted to have antithrombotic properties.[22,23] In addition, HCQ favorably alters lipid profiles, which may be of use in RA patients in view of their increased risk of cardiovascular disease.[24] The primary toxicity of this medication is ophthalmologic, secondary to deposition of pigment in the retina, and routine monitoring by an ophthalmologist is required to detect this rare complication before permanent damage occurs. The dose of HCQ should never exceed 6.5 mg/kg/d to best avoid retinal toxicity.

Sulfasalazine is another, older DMARD that also has proven benefit for RA patients with relatively

Table 1
Common treatments for rheumatoid arthritis, and their targets and toxicities

Conventional DMARDs	Target	Testing Before Starting Medication	Toxicities	Monitoring
Methotrexate	Enhances adenosine release; inhibits polyamines; folic acid antagonist	Cr, CBC, LFTs, hepatitis B and C screening	Nausea, diarrhea, liver toxicity, pneumonitis, cytopenias, infections, lymphoma	LFTs, Cr, CBC every 4–8 wk
Leflunomide	Pyrimidine synthesis	Cr, CBC, LFTs, hepatitis B and C screening	Nausea, diarrhea, liver toxicity, pneumonitis (rare), infections	LFTs, Cr, CBC every 4–8 wk
Hydroxychloroquine	TLR signaling; stabilization of lysosomal membranes	Retinal screen	Retinal toxicity, nausea	Yearly ophthalmologic examination
Sulfasalazine	Enhances adenosine pathways and inhibits arachidonic acid	CBC	Nausea, diarrhea, allergic reactions, neutropenia (rare)	CBC every 4–8 wk during first year of treatment
Biologic DMARDs				
Anti-TNF drugs	TNF-α	TB screen, hepatitis B and C screen, fungal screens (depending on geography)	Infusion and injection site reactions, rash, infections, lymphoma	None
Rituximab	CD-20	Hepatitis B screen, TB screen	Infusion reaction (can be severe), PML (rare)	None
Abatacept	CTLA-4 CD 80/86 interaction	TB screen, hepatitis B and C screen, fungal screens (depending on geography)	Possible infusion reaction, infections	None
Anakinra	IL-1 receptor antagonist	TB screen, CBC	Injection site reactions, neutropenia, infections	Monthly CBC
Tocilizumab	IL-6 receptor antagonist	Lipid profile, CBC, TB screen, hepatitis B and C screen, fungal screens (depending on geography)	Neutropenia, thrombocytopenia, elevated total cholesterol and triglycerides, bowel perforations (rare), infections	Monthly CBC, Cr, cholesterol profile

Abbreviations: CBC, complete blood count; Cr, creatinine; IL, interleukin; LFTs, liver function tests; PML, progressive multifocal leukoencephalopathy; TB, tuberculosis; TLR, toll-like receptor; TNF, tumor necrosis factor.

low toxicity. Similar to methotrexate, it enhances adenosine signaling and may also inhibit arachidonic acid pathways. Placebo-controlled studies have shown improvement in pain and function within 4 weeks of treatment with sulfasalazine. In addition, sulfasalazine has been shown to slow radiographic progression after 1 to 3 years of therapy.[20,25] However, it is generally considered a less potent DMARD and is typically used as part of a combination regimen. Gastrointestinal distress is the primary side effect of sulfasalazine, although allergic reactions and rashes may preclude its use. Leukopenia, which can be severe, occurs rarely during the first year of sulfasalazine treatment.

Other medications such as azathioprine, minocycline, doxycycline, and cyclosporine have all been shown to have beneficial effects on disease activity in RA, but are typically used as adjunctive or substitute medications when the other DMARDs cannot be used secondary to adverse reactions. Injectable gold salts are an older form of treatment that can slow radiographic progression even without a full clinical response.[20] However, with the advent of more reliable, less toxic medications, injectable gold has almost disappeared as a DMARD for RA.

Biologic DMARDs

The availability of medications targeted toward specific abnormalities of the immune system, the so-called biologic DMARDs, has revolutionized the treatment of RA. This expanding collection of drugs targets molecules that have been shown to play important roles in the pathology of RA. Because of their cost and side effect profile, the use of biologic DMARDs is typically recommended after patients have failed the use of single or combination conventional DMARD therapy. However, in patients who present with highly aggressive, erosive disease, they can be considered as a component of first-line therapy. Biologic DMARDs typically are not used in combination with each other, but trials are ongoing to evaluate the risks and benefits of combination therapy between different biologic DMARD classes.

The initial choice of a biologic DMARD is typically a TNF blocking agent, which includes infliximab, adulimumab, etanercept, and the newer golimumab and certolizumab. These agents have varied effects on a molecular level including binding soluble $TNF\alpha$ and induction of apoptosis of $TNF\alpha$-expressing cells. Each of these drugs has a distinct dosing schedule or mode of administration. However, all appear to have similar benefits in RA.[26] These agents work more rapidly than nonbiologic DMARDs, with responses often seen within

4 to 8 weeks, occasionally earlier. All are effective as monotherapy, but have significantly more benefit on clinical response and prevention of radiographic progression if used in conjunction with a DMARD such as methotrexate.[27] However, the combination of anti-TNF therapy and methotrexate is not more effective for the clinical manifestations of RA than a combination of conventional DMARDs (methotrexate+sulfasalazine+HCQ).[17] Prolonged follow-up to compare effectiveness at a structural level as monitored by serial radiographs is ongoing. Despite the success of anti-TNF medications, up to 30% of patients with RA may not have a clinical response to anti-TNF therapy.[28] However, these medications have been shown to slow and/or inhibit radiographic progression in RA patients, even without other evidence of clinical improvement.[19,26] Some patients benefit from switching from one anti-TNF medication to another, but failure of multiple TNF inhibitors to improve symptoms often leads to the use of other biologic DMARD medications.[26]

The evidence for the role of B cells in the pathogenesis of RA is increasing rapidly. The recruitment of B cells to inflamed synovium and the production of inflammatory cytokines that stimulate osteoclasts suggest an important role for this cell type in the etiology of RA.[29] Rituximab is a chimeric anti-CD20 monoclonal antibody that depletes immature and mature B cells, but not plasma cells, which lack CD20 expression. Rituximab is approved for moderate to severe RA in patients who do not have adequate response to conventional DMARDs and anti-TNF medications.[19] A recent randomized, placebo-controlled trial of rituximab showed that when used in conjunction with methotrexate, rituximab slows radiographic progression after a year of treatment.[30] A sustained response appears possible with intermittent courses of treatment that consist of 2 intravenous infusions given 2 weeks apart, and repeated every 6 months before the return of symptoms.[31] Serious infusion reactions can occur, which are often avoided by including intravenous methylprednisolone with the pr-infusion medications.

Abatacept is a fusion protein of cytotoxic T-lymphocyte—associated antigen 4 (CTLA-4) and the Fc portion of IgG1. Abatacept interferes with the interaction of CD80/CD86 molecules on antigen-presenting cells with their receptor CD28, a molecule on the T-cell surface that normally senses the "second signal" required for T-cell activation. This process results in decreased T-cell activation and ultimately decreased joint inflammation. Abatacept is currently recommended for treatment of RA after a trial of conventional DMARD therapy or an anti-TNF agent has failed to induce acceptable disease improvement.[19] Although the onset of efficacy is slower than some of the other biologic medications, treatment with abatacept provides persistent improvement in disease activity and radiographic progression.[28,32] In addition, unlike other biologic DMARDs, some research suggests that abatacept may not increase serious infection risk over that seen with nonbiologic DMARDs, which may make it a more appealing option in patients more prone to infectious complications.[33]

Anakinra, an IL-1 receptor antagonist, has been approved as a second-line treatment for RA after failure of another biologic DMARD, typically an anti-TNF medication. In Europe, its use is recommended in conjunction with methotrexate.[19] Daily injections have been shown to improve patient function and radiographic progression; however, this effect is less than the improvements seen with anti-TNF therapy.[34] Anakinra has at most a limited role in the treatment of RA, although it has important benefits in rare systemic febrile inflammatory syndromes such as pediatric and adult Still disease (for which it is not currently approved by the Food and Drug Administration).

Tocilizumab is a recently approved biologic therapy for moderate to severe RA. Tocilizumab is a recombinant humanized monoclonal antibody that binds to the IL-6 receptor. IL-6 is a proinflammatory cytokine that is increased in the serum of RA patients. Monthly infusions of tocilizumab improve function and quality of life, and slow radiographic progression in patients who have failed management with traditional DMARDs or anti-TNF therapy.[35,36] This effect of tocilizumab is greater when it is used in conjunction with methotrexate.[36] Its unique mechanism of action is associated with an increased risk of elevated liver enzymes and a reversible elevation in total cholesterol and triglycerides, thus appropriate selection of patients is important for this medication.[36] Transient neutropenia and thrombocytopenia can be seen in 1% to 3% of patients after infusion, and intestinal perforations have also been noted.[36]

COMPLICATIONS OF MEDICAL TREATMENT OF RA

RA itself confers an elevated risk of infection, and DMARD and biologic therapies suppress the immune system through various targets, which also increases this risk.[37] Bacterial infections, particularly pneumonia and soft-tissue infections, are increased with the use of methotrexate, and this is increased 2- to 4-fold with the addition of an anti-TNF medication.[38] Similar infectious risks have been found with other biologic DMARDs as well.[28,35] A significant risk of reactivation of tuberculosis (TB) has also been noted with anti-TNF medication.[39] Thus, screening for TB exposure and treatment of latent TB before initiation of anti-TNF agents is recommended. Similar precautions are in place for other RA biologics, although the actual risk of TB due to these medications is less well understood. TNF blockers also increase the risk for severe and systemic fungal infections such as histoplasmosis and coccidioidomycosis, which may be a significant issue in specific geographic locales. An increased risk of viral infections with traditional or biologic DMARDs, including varicella zoster virus, Epstein-Barr virus, and cytomegalovirus has been documented.[40] Hepatitis B and C reactivation have also occurred with biologic DMARDs, so screening before treatment and vaccination when possible is recommended.[40,41] Progressive multifocal leukoencephalopathy, an infection caused by reactivation of the JC virus, has also been reported in RA patients treated with rituximab.[42]

Immunosuppression also can lead to a theoretical risk of malignancy, as tumor surveillance by the immune system may be affected. Because RA patients have an increased risk of lymphoma secondary to the disease itself, the extent of the increased risk of developing a cancer such as lymphoma while taking immunosuppressive medications remains debatable.[43] A recent analysis of a German RA registry did not find an increased risk of malignancy, either hematologic or solid tumor, with the use of anti-TNF agents or anakinra; however, this included only 4 years of exposure data.[44] By contrast, an analysis of French patients on anti-TNF medications has shown an increased incidence of lymphoma in patients on adalimumab or infliximab.[45] The coexistence of other autoimmune diseases, such as Sjögren syndrome, may also increase the likelihood of developing lymphoma, thus making it more difficult to determine the contribution from immunosuppressive medications.[45]

PERIOPERATIVE MANAGEMENT

Because of the nature of their disease, patients with RA have many features that can affect perioperative management. Thus, consultation with a patient's rheumatologist prior to surgery may help to identify unique risks for that patient and prevent perioperative morbidity and mortality.

Given their elevated cardiac risk factors, a thorough cardiovascular history and physical examination should be completed in all RA patients before surgery. Depending on their risk profile and activity level, either an exercise or pharmacologic stress test could be considered to stratify their risk for cardiovascular complications. In addition, patients with risk factors for interstitial lung disease, such as seropositivity (positive rheumatoid factor and/or positive titer of antibodies to citrulline-containing proteins), smoking, chronic cough, or complaints of shortness of breath should have pulmonary function testing completed before surgery, thus allowing for maximization of lung function before anesthesia.

Cervical spine involvement is common in RA and it parallels the progression of peripheral joint erosions, especially of the hands and feet.[46] Thus, patients considering hand surgery for RA complications should be screened for cervical disease. In RA, the alignment of the cervical spine can be compromised secondary to joint erosions or ligamentous laxity from synovial inflammation. This process leads to anterior, posterior, or vertical subluxation, and if severe can result in spinal cord and/or brainstem injury or even death with neck manipulation, such as during intubation. Symptoms of cervical instability include neck pain that radiates to the occiput, painless sensory loss in the hands, changes in consciousness with head motion, difficulty walking that is unexplained by RA involvement of the lower extremity joints, or paresthesias of the shoulders or arms with head motion. However, subluxation can be asymptomatic in as many as 31% of patients, so a screening cervical spine series that includes additional lateral views in both flexion and extension should be considered in all patients who will require intubation.[46] Significant abnormalities noted on plain radiographs should prompt a neurosurgical consult as well as a preoperative MRI with contrast to assess the existence or threat of injury to the spinal cord.

The medications used to treat RA also provide for challenges in the perioperative period. Many patients with RA use chronic, low-dose steroids to improve their daily function. As a result, these patients must be assumed to have a suppressed hypothalamic-pituitary-adrenal (HPA) axis and thus be prone to adrenal insufficiency in times of stress, such as surgery or infection. Current guidelines suggest that any patient receiving more than 5 mg of prednisone per day should receive higher dose replacement during the perioperative period.[47] Minor noninvasive procedures, such as outpatient hand surgery, may not require steroid supplementation.[48] However, any procedure that requires general anesthesia should be considered more invasive and these patients should be given intravenous hydrocortisone, 50 to 100 mg preoperatively and possibly additional intravenous steroid doses over the subsequent 24-hour period before resuming their usual oral steroid dose. Severely ill patients or those who undergo extreme procedures such as cardiothoracic surgery should have their stress dose of hydrocortisone tapered by half every day postoperatively until they reach their maintenance dose.[47,48] For patients who have recently been on steroid treatment in whom the status of their HPA axis is unclear, an adrenocorticotropic hormone stimulation test may highlight patients whose endogenous steroid production would be suppressed under stress and thus would benefit from steroid supplementation perioperatively.

RA patients have an increased risk of infection after orthopedic surgery.[49] The use of DMARDs and biologic DMARDs can increase the risk of infection and theoretically may impair wound healing. There is ongoing debate regarding which medications to interrupt perioperatively. Current recommendations for perioperative use of these medications are summarized in **Table 2**. Although some studies suggest that it is safe to continue using methotrexate through surgery, a prudent recommendation is to hold the doses before and immediately after surgery.[50] Plaquenil has a long half-life and does not confer an increased risk of infection, thus its use is typically continued in the perioperative period. Sulfasalazine may be continued without interruption other than on the day of surgery. Leflunomide should be held at least 1 week before surgery, although more data are needed to guide recommendations regarding this medication, in view of its especially long half-life.

Anti-TNF agents have been sparsely studied with regard to their perioperative use. There is a theoretical risk of increased susceptibility to gram-positive infections but there are no definitive data for this. In fact most studies, including those that examined surgical procedures on small joints, have not found an increased risk of wound infections with concomitant use of anti-TNF agents.[37] No data exist as to their effects on wound healing. Because of the paucity of data, a reasonable approach is to hold anti-TNF medications for one dosage cycle perioperatively. Postoperative complications such as wound infection should delay resumption of anti-TNF agents, methotrexate, leflunomide, or other cytotoxic/immunosuppressive agents.

Other biologic medications with longer half-lives make the timing of surgery even more uncertain. Rituximab can result in B-cell depletion for up to 6 months, albeit without profound hypogammaglobulinemia. Elective surgery is probably safest when B-cell counts have rebounded. The half-life of abatacept is 15 days, so holding this medication

Table 2
Perioperative management of medications used to treat RA

Medication	Perioperative Management
Steroids	Continue at lowest dose possible; consider stress dose steroids as indicated
Methotrexate	Hold doses immediately before and after surgery
Leflunomide	Hold at least 1 week before surgery[a]
Hydroxychloroquine	Continue perioperatively
Sulfasalazine	Hold only on day of surgery
Anti-TNF drugs	Hold for one dose perioperatively
Rituximab	Optimal timing of surgery when CD20 counts have rebounded (3–6 months after last dose)
Abatacept	Hold 1 month before surgery
Anakinra	Hold 1 week before and after surgery[a]
Tocilizumab	Hold dose before surgery[a]

[a] More evidence is needed to affirm recommendation.

for 1 month before surgery is reasonable.[37] Data regarding the use of tocilizumab in the perioperative period are minimal, but it has been shown to suppress postoperative fever and cause an increase in inflammatory markers.[37] Thus, holding it in the perioperative period would also be a reasonable approach.

SUMMARY

RA is a common disease with widespread focal joint destruction and complications secondary to systemic inflammation. Recent treatment options based on better understanding of disease pathology have led to immense changes in the management of this disease. The aggressive use of DMARDs and biologic DMARD therapy has allowed patients to achieve improved function and decreased joint destruction. These medications are not without side effects or long-term risks, however. An understanding of these pitfalls will allow for optimal patient care in both the medical and surgical settings.

REFERENCES

1. Vosse D, de Vlam K. Osteoporosis in rheumatoid arthritis and ankylosing spondylitis. Clin Exp Rheumatol 2009;27:S62.
2. Gravallese E, Harada Y, Wang J, et al. Identification of cell types responsible for bone resorption in rheumatoid arthritis and juvenile rheumatoid arthritis. Am J Pathol 1998;152:943.
3. Walsh NC, Reinwald S, Manning CA, et al. Osteoblast function is compromised at sites of focal bone erosion in inflammatory arthritis. J Bone Miner Res 2009;24:1572.
4. Ideguchi H, Ohno S, Hattori H, et al. Bone erosions in rheumatoid arthritis can be repaired through reduction in disease activity with conventional disease-modifying antirheumatic drugs. Arthritis Res Ther 2006;8:R76.
5. Sinigaglia L, Nervetti A, Mela Q, et al. A multicenter cross sectional study on bone mineral density in rheumatoid arthritis. Italian study group on bone mass in rheumatoid arthritis. J Rheumatol 2000;27:2582.
6. El Maghraoui A, Rezqi A, Mounach A, et al. Prevalence and risk factors of vertebral fractures in women with rheumatoid arthritis using vertebral fracture assessment. Rheumatology 2010;49(7):1303–10.
7. Matos M, Tannuri U, Guarniero R. The effect of zoledronate during bone healing. J Orthop Traumatol 2010;11:7.
8. Devouassoux G, Cottin V, Liote H, et al. Characterisation of severe obliterative bronchiolitis in rheumatoid arthritis. Eur Respir J 2009;33:1053.
9. Kelly C, Saravanan V. Treatment strategies for a rheumatoid arthritis patient with interstitial lung disease. Expert Opin Pharmacother 2008;9:3221.
10. Mori S, Cho I, Koga Y, et al. A simultaneous onset of organizing pneumonia and rheumatoid arthritis, along with a review of the literature. Mod Rheumatol 2008;18:60.
11. Radovits BJ, Fransen J, Shamma SA, et al. Excess mortality emerges after 10 years in an inception cohort of early rheumatoid arthritis. Arthritis Care Res 2010;62:362.
12. Peters MJL, VPv Halm, Voskuyl AE, et al. Does rheumatoid arthritis equal diabetes mellitus as an independent risk factor for cardiovascular disease? A prospective study. Arthritis Care Res 2009;61:1571.
13. Bergholm R, Leirisalo-Repo M, Vehkavaara S, et al. Impaired responsiveness to NO in newly diagnosed

patients with rheumatoid arthritis. Arterioscler Thromb Vasc Biol 2002;22:1637.

14. Maradit-Kremers H, Nicola PJ, Crowson CS, et al. Cardiovascular death in rheumatoid arthritis: a population-based study. Arthritis Rheum 2005;52:722.

15. Verstappen SMM, Jacobs JWG, Bijlsma JWJ, et al. Five-year followup of rheumatoid arthritis patients after early treatment with disease-modifying antirheumatic drugs versus treatment according to the pyramid approach in the first year. Arthritis Rheum 2003;48:1797.

16. Weng HH, Ranganath VK, Khanna D, et al. Equivalent responses to disease-modifying antirheumatic drugs initiated at any time during the first 15 months after symptom onset in patients with seropositive rheumatoid arthritis. J Rheumatol 2010;37:550.

17. Ma MHY, Kingsley GH, Scott DL. A systematic comparison of combination DMARD therapy and tumour necrosis inhibitor therapy with methotrexate in patients with early rheumatoid arthritis. Rheumatology 2010;49:91.

18. Chan ESL, Cronstein B. Methotrexate—how does it really work? Nat Rev Rheumatol 2010;6:175.

19. Furst DE, Breedveld FC, Kalden JR, et al. Updated consensus statement on biological agents for the treatment of rheumatic diseases, 2009. Ann Rheum Dis 2010;69(Suppl 1):i2–29.

20. Pincus T, Ferraccioli G, Sokka T, et al. Evidence from clinical trials and long-term observational studies that disease-modifying anti-rheumatic drugs slow radiographic progression in rheumatoid arthritis: updating a 1983 review. Rheumatology 2002;41:1346.

21. Strand V, Cohen S, Schiff M, et al. Treatment of active rheumatoid arthritis with leflunomide compared with placebo and methotrexate. Arch Intern Med 1999;159:2542.

22. Ruiz-Irastorza G, Egurbide MV, Pijoan JI, et al. Effect of antimalarials on thrombosis and survival in patients with systemic lupus erythematosus. Lupus 2006;15:577.

23. Wasko MCM, Hubert H, Lingala V, et al. Hydroxychloroquine and risk of diabetes in patients with rheumatoid arthritis. JAMA 2007;298:187.

24. Tam LS, Gladman DD, Hallett DC, et al. Effect of antimalarial agents on the fasting lipid profile in systemic lupus erythematosus. J Rheumatol 2000;27:2142.

25. Hannonen P, Möttönen T, Hakola M, et al. Sulfasalazine in early rheumatoid arthritis. A 48-week double-blind, prospective, placebo-controlled study. Arthritis Rheum 1993;36:1501.

26. Statkute L, Ruderman EM. Novel TNF antagonists for the treatment of rheumatoid arthritis. Expert Opin Investig Drugs 2010;19:105.

27. Breedveld FC, Weisman MH, Kavanaugh AF, et al. The PREMIER study: a multicenter, randomized, double-blind clinical trial of combination therapy with adalimumab plus methotrexate versus methotrexate alone or adalimumab alone in patients with early, aggressive rheumatoid arthritis who had not had previous methotrexate treatment. Arthritis Rheum 2006;54:26.

28. Genovese MC, Schiff M, Luggen M, et al. Efficacy and safety of the selective co-stimulation modulator abatacept following 2 years of treatment in patients with rheumatoid arthritis and an inadequate response to anti-tumour necrosis factor therapy. Ann Rheum Dis 2008;67:547.

29. Marston B, Palanichamy A, Anolik JH. B cells in the pathogenesis and treatment of rheumatoid arthritis. Curr Opin Rheumatol 2010;22:307.

30. Keystone E, Emery P, Peterfy CG, et al. Rituximab inhibits structural joint damage in patients with rheumatoid arthritis with an inadequate response to tumour necrosis factor inhibitor therapies. Ann Rheum Dis 2009;68:216.

31. Mease PJ, Cohen S, Gaylis NB, et al. Efficacy and safety of retreatment in patients with rheumatoid arthritis with previous inadequate response to tumor necrosis factor inhibitors: results from the SUNRISE trial. J Rheumatol 2010;37.

32. Kremer JM, Genant HK, Moreland LW, et al. Results of a two-year followup study of patients with rheumatoid arthritis who received a combination of abatacept and methotrexate. Arthritis Rheum 2008;58:953.

33. Simon T, Askling J, Lacaille D, et al. Infections requiring hospitalization in the Abatacept clinical development program: an epidemiological assessment. Arthritis Res Ther 2010;12:R67.

34. Mertens M, Singh JA. Anakinra for rheumatoid arthritis. Cochrane Database Syst Rev 2009;1:CD005121.

35. Emery P, Keystone E, Tony HP, et al. IL-6 receptor inhibition with tocilizumab improves treatment outcomes in patients with rheumatoid arthritis refractory to anti-tumour necrosis factor biologicals: results from a 24-week multicentre randomised placebo-controlled trial. Ann Rheum Dis 2008;67:1516.

36. Oldfield V, Dhillon S, Plosker GL. Tocilizumab: a review of its use in the management of rheumatoid arthritis. Drugs 2009;69:609.

37. Mushtaq S, Goodman SM, Scanzello CR. Perioperative management of biologic agents used in treatment of rheumatoid arthritis. Am J Ther 2010 [online].

38. Curtis JR, Patkar N, Xie A, et al. Risk of serious bacterial infections among rheumatoid arthritis patients exposed to tumor necrosis factor alpha antagonists. Arthritis Rheum 2007;56:1125.

39. Dixon WG, Hyrich KL, Watson KD, et al. Drug-specific risk of tuberculosis in patients with rheumatoid arthritis treated with anti-TNF therapy: results from the British Society for Rheumatology Biologics Register (BSRBR). Ann Rheum Dis 2010;69:522.

40. Kim SY, Solomon DH. Tumor necrosis factor blockade and the risk of viral infection. Nat Rev Rheumatol 2010;6:165.

41. Roux CH, Brocq O, Breuil V, et al. Safety of anti-TNF-{alpha} therapy in rheumatoid arthritis and spondylarthropathies with concurrent B or C chronic hepatitis. Rheumatology 2006;45:1294.

42. Fleischmann RM. Progressive multifocal leukoencephalopathy following rituximab treatment in a patient with rheumatoid arthritis. Arthritis Rheum 2009;60: 3225.

43. Askling JA, Bongartz TB. Malignancy and biologic therapy in rheumatoid arthritis. Curr Opin Rheumatol 2008;20:334.

44. Strangfeld A, Hierse F, Rau R, et al. Risk of incident or recurrent malignancies among patients with rheumatoid arthritis exposed to biologic therapy in the German biologics register RABBIT. Arthritis Res Ther 2010;12:R5.

45. Mariette X, Tubach F, Bagheri H, et al. Lymphoma in patients treated with anti-TNF: results of the 3-year prospective French RATIO registry. Ann Rheum Dis 2010;69:400.

46. Neva MH, Häkkinen A, Mäkinen H, et al. High prevalence of asymptomatic cervical spine subluxation in patients with rheumatoid arthritis waiting for orthopaedic surgery. Ann Rheum Dis 2006;65:884.

47. Coursin DB, Wood KE. Corticosteroid supplementation for adrenal insufficiency. JAMA 2002;287:236.

48. Fleager K, Yao J. Perioperative steroid dosing in patients receiving chronic oral steroids, undergoing outpatient hand surgery. J Hand Surg 2010;35:316.

49. Bongartz T, Halligan CS, Osmon DR, et al. Incidence and risk factors of prosthetic joint infection after total hip or knee replacement in patients with rheumatoid arthritis. Arthritis Care Res 2008;59:1713.

50. Pieringer H, Stuby U, Biesenbach G. The place of methotrexate perioperatively in elective orthopedic surgeries in patients with rheumatoid arthritis. Clin Rheumatol 2008;27:1217.

Controversy in the Surgical Treatment of the Rheumatoid Hand

Ronald J. Anderson, MD[a,b,*]

KEYWORDS

- Rheumatoid arthritis • Hand • Treatment • Intervention

The clinical picture of rheumatoid arthritis (RA) is best viewed as a combination of systemic symptoms associated with the inflammatory process and articular symptoms related both to potentially reversible synovitis and structural damage brought on by inflammation. In simple terms, the treatment of inflammation is medical, and structural lesions often require surgical solutions.

The course of RA is marked by its persistence. Spontaneous remissions are rare and usually occur only in the first year of the disease.[1] Although the effectiveness of antiinflammatory therapies has improved greatly in the last decade, their action is more likely to suppress rather than eliminate structural damage. Most patients with RA develop some structural damage during the course of their disease, and more than half the patients may anticipate undergoing a reconstructive procedure.[2] However, in any given patient with RA, it is rare to have all joints involved, and frequently only a few joints are affected. Evidence exists indicating that virtually all of the joints that ultimately become involved in a given patient with RA are evident on physical examination during the first year of the disease.[3] Therefore, given the worse case scenario that the disease remains active, one can usually predict which joints will ultimately become damaged and which will not.

Advances in the reconstructive management of RA in the last several decades have been considerable and have virtually eliminated the fear of major crippling problems related to the disease.

However, the appropriate orchestration and selection of surgical interventions are both controversial and problematic for the physician involved in the care of these patients. The discordance between surgeons and rheumatologists about the value and indications for surgical intervention has been well documented.[4] Surgical literature focuses primarily on the technical aspects of the procedures and descriptions of complications. Randomized controlled studies of surgical versus nonsurgical interventions do not exist. There is little published on the comparative efficacy of alternative procedures and virtually nothing on the role of a single procedure in the total surgical care of the patient with involvement of multiple joints. In addition, there is little long-term follow-up on the results and complications of these procedures, which is a major issue in decision making for the care of patients with a chronic disease such as RA.

PRINCIPLES OF SURGICAL INTERVENTION

The prime indications for surgery in patients with RA are essentially determined by the patient and consist of a desire to obtain pain relief and/or functional improvement.[5] Pain is difficult to quantify. However, it is useful to define pain according to whether it is severe enough to alter sleep. In most situations, pain sufficient to alter sleep is an indication for surgical repair. Symptoms producing nocturnal pain associated with structural damage are rare in the hand, and, when present, are

[a] Division of Rheumatology, Immunology and Allergy, Brigham and Women's Hospital, Boston, MA 02115, USA
[b] Harvard Medical School, Boston, MA, USA
* Corresponding author. Division of Rheumatology, Immunology and Allergy, Brigham and Women's Hospital, Boston, MA 02115.
E-mail address: randerson@partners.org

Hand Clin 27 (2011) 21–25
doi:10.1016/j.hcl.2010.10.007
0749-0712/11/$ — see front matter © 2011 Elsevier Inc. All rights reserved.

more likely related to an associated carpal tunnel syndrome. This syndrome is more commonly seen early in the course of RA. This observation is presumably because the retinaculum holding in the synovium of the wrist has not been stretched and distended early in the course of the disease. The confined spaces create greater pressure within both the wrist and the carpal tunnel. These patients usually respond to conservative interventions such as splinting or local injection with steroids.

Evaluating the potential for functional gain is more involved, and the physician must be aware of other limitations that would be uncovered by significant improvement in the worse joint. This possibility is more likely to be an issue in the decision to operate on the lower extremity. For example, when contemplating a total hip replacement for an individual with RA who is comfortable at rest but experiences right hip pain after walking 1 block, the possibility that the patient's left knee will become symptomatic after walking 2 blocks or that angina will develop after walking 3 blocks should be explored.

Cosmetic concerns also play a significant role in the decision to advise hand surgery, but are seldom a consideration in surgery on any other joints. Similarly to the face, the appearance of the hand is critical to many individuals' self-image. Shaking hands and other activities using the hand are essential parts of interpersonal interaction. The question of cosmetic goals is seldom included in protocols used to evaluate hand surgery. However, it may be the major issue that determines the level of a patient's satisfaction with a procedure. It is imperative to inquire about and frankly discuss cosmetic goals with a patient who is considering operative intervention on the hand. Although it has great meaning to them, patients with RA may be embarrassed and reluctant to discuss it openly.

Therapeutic interventions available to patients with RA are shown in **Box 1**. Synovectomies and tenosynovectomies involve debridement of inflammatory tissue and are predominantly intended to prevent further damage to the tendons or the joints. The articular surfaces are left intact and all options are kept open. Reconstructive procedures that create an irreversible alteration of the articular anatomy are performed in individuals in whom the cartilage has been significantly destroyed.

ESSENTIAL CONCEPTS REGARDING SURGICAL INTERVENTIONS IN RA
Surgery is Elective

The ultimate result obtained from a surgical intervention is usually independent of the timing of the operation. However, the physician should encourage the repair of a destroyed or dysfunctional joint when the damage significantly impedes critical function to the point that potential loss of social or economic independence is threatened. This outcome is an issue predominantly in joints of the lower extremity in which mobility is at risk, and seldom is a factor in the hand. However, there are a few situations in which an absolute indication for immediate (within the next few days) surgery exists in patients with RA.

Instability of the cervical spine with resultant myelopathy and neurologic damage

This complication is often heralded by progressive weakness that cannot be explained by other mechanisms. Bilateral hand paresthesias are often seen, most commonly in the ulnar distribution of the hand. Accentuated neck pain does not characteristically accompany this lesion and may even be absent.

Rupture of the ulnar extensor tendons at the wrist

This lesion may result from an extensor tenosynovitis of the dorsum of the wrist, but more frequently is related to an attrition rupture. This injury occurs when the long, ring, and little extensor tendons are abraded by the sawtooth surface of an ulnar styloid that has been eroded by persistent synovitis. The rupture usually first occurs in the little finger extensor and may be asymptomatic because pain is seldom an issue; inability to extend the little finger may not be lost because a tendinous slip often attaches the ring to the little finger extensor tendon that allows the ring finger to extend the little finger. On physical examination, this may be detected by observing the inability of the little finger to extend when the ring finger is held in flexion at the metacarpophalangeal (MCP) joint. Surgery is indicated not only to attempt a repair of the ruptured tendon, but, more importantly, to remove the distal ulna and thus prevent further ruptures to the ring or long fingers.

Box 1
Orthopedic procedures in the treatment of RA

Prophylactic and therapeutic

    Synovectomy

    Tenosynovectomy

Therapeutic

    Resection arthroplasty

    Arthrodesis

    Total joint replacement

Removal of the prosthesis from an infected joint

In most situations, the prosthetic elements are removed and antibiotics continued for a prolonged period of time before attempting to reinsert a new prosthesis. The functional limitations associated with this waiting period are more severe in a lower extremity joint than in the hand, in which, with the exception of removal of a total wrist prosthesis, absence of the missing prosthesis is better tolerated.

Surgery is Local Therapy

Surgical procedures cannot be evaluated in isolation and must be viewed both in relation to adjacent joints and in regard to the patient as a whole. These factors should be considered when selecting surgical interventions. Some procedures are more effective than others. The tendency of many surgeons to limit their procedures to a specific region may limit their viewpoint and argues strongly that the surgical management of patients with RA should be orchestrated by a knowledgeable rheumatologist or another competent physician who has a global perspective of the patient.

Other considerations are the amount of energy expended, anesthetic risk, and temporary disability (downtime) associated with the procedure itself. For many patients, the critical question is not "Will the operation help?" but "Is it worth the effort?" A patient's ultimate attitude toward further surgery is often based on his or her experience with initial surgical procedures. For these reasons, it is important in the management of a patient who will require multiple procedures to advise an initial operation with the highest likelihood of success. In simple terms: lead with a winner.

WHAT IS UNIQUE ABOUT THE HAND IN RA COMPARED WITH OTHER JOINTS?

Given the worst possible case scenario of an unrelenting destructive inflammatory process involving all the joints of the hand, what can be expected both symptomatically and functionally without surgical intervention? Biomechanically, the wrist is the major weight-bearing joint of the hand and the one most likely to experience pain when grasping is performed. In making a fist, the forearm musculature affects the hand on the forearm at the wrist. The MCP joints bear little weight and, if the characteristic subluxations associated with joint destruction occur, the joint becomes even more non—weight bearing and rarely evolves as a source of pain. Although it is optimal to have the use of all 5 fingers, the critical functions of the fingers are dependent on having an opposable

thumb and a stable index finger, which allows an individual to pinch.

In summary, the goals of any treatment of the hand should be focused on providing a wrist that is able to sustain the forces of grasping without disabling pain, and having thumb and index finger that are stable and able to oppose each other with a functional pinch.

EFFICACY OF, AND INDICATIONS FOR, SPECIFIC SURGICAL PROCEDURES ON THE HAND IN PATIENTS WITH RA

The reader should now be warned that we are entering a data-free zone. For the reasons mentioned previously, critical analysis of the relative effectiveness of different procedures is lacking in the literature and data on the comparative value of different procedures in a given patient with RA are essentially nonexistent. The concepts and views expressed in this article are based on literature review and almost 40 years of experience as a clinical rheumatologist at the Brigham and Women's Hospital. The rheumatologists in our hospital have always worked across the hall from the surgeons, and this has provided a unique opportunity to work in an integrated and cooperative manner with a talented group of surgeons and rheumatologists, and a chance to follow a large group of patients with this difficult disease for an extended period of time. It has also been my custom over the years to ask patients with RA, particularly those who have had multiple procedures, to rate the different operations. Another useful technique for the evaluation of the value of specific procedures on a limb is to ascertain the frequency with which the patient elects to have the other side done after the first procedure has healed.

Synovectomies and Tenosynovectomies

The examination of the hand should always include an examination of the tendons. The observation of any discrepancy between active and passive motion indicates that the problem does not lie with the joint but with the tendons, the muscles, or the nerves. Palpation of the palm while having the patient actively flex and extend the fingers indicates the presence of nodules and/or flexor tenosynovitis. Extensor tenosynovitis is also commonly seen in RA but is more evident to both the patient and the untrained observer. These conditions are present in virtually all patients with RA and may be dominant complaints at various times during the course of the disease. Tendon nodules, like rheumatoid nodules elsewhere, tend to recede in size with time, and frequently disappear. Obstructing nodules most often respond to a local steroid injection into the sheath, and surgical repair is seldom required. The concept that the process is potentially reversible, either by medical intervention or natural course, should be the guiding principle. For these reasons, surgical correction of obstructing nodules is seldom indicated and management by medical therapy, maintenance of passive range of motion, and occasional local injection is usually sufficient.

Tendon ruptures related to erosive tenosynovitis may occur, although rarely. This is the basis used to advocate prophylactic tenosynovectomies intended to avoid future tendon ruptures. Arguments against this approach are:

1. Essentially all patients with RA have tenosynovitis. If tenosynovectomies were used on all these individuals, neither the patients nor the surgeons would have time for much else in their lives.
2. Most tendon ruptures are attrition ruptures related primarily to erosive damage that creates a sawtooth edge on the ulnar styloid.
3. Rupture of the extensor pollicis longus seems to be the most common tendon rupture in RA related to tenosynovitis. Many patients with this lesion are able to compensate for the loss of power in extension of the thumb interphalangeal (IP) joint with the extensor pollicus brevis and choose not to have the repair because their functional loss is not a significant problem for them.

Synovectomy in RA, particularly of the wrist, has a theoretic appeal without a strong track record. In recent years, perhaps related to improvements in the medical management of the disease, there seem to be fewer advocates of this procedure. The general experience has been that the process returns in a few years and the effort expended on a single joint is not worthwhile in a systemic disease. However, there are arguments for combining a synovectomy with another procedure. For example, when the ulnar head is being resected related to an attrition rupture, including a wrist synovectomy makes sense. Another condition is to perform an elbow synovectomy in conjunction with a radial head excision or ulnar nerve transposition.

Joint Arthroplasties

Arthroplasties involving the hand may be classified as fusions, resection arthroplasties, or total joint replacements. The silicone MCP implant arthroplasty is an interpositional arthroplasty rather than a total joint replacement, because the silicone implant is not wedded to the bone but acts as a spacer. The procedure is unique and can only be used in a fundamentally non—weight-bearing joint.

Wrist Procedures

Pain leading to significant dysfunction is the indication for considering a procedure on the rheumatoid wrist: either fusion or total wrist arthroplasty. In making a decision about the type of procedure to have, patients tend to be hesitant about selecting a wrist fusion, envisioning increased immobility and further loss of function. The total wrist arthroplasty has the appeal of possibly restoring what has been lost anatomically. Few of the patients considering wrist arthroplasty have more than 10 to 20 degrees of total wrist motion, and the decreased motion is seldom related to pain. There is concern about the long-term viability of total wrist arthroplasties. A 17% removal rate of the implant at 8 years may be viewed as excessive[6] and one report describes a need for revision in most patients.[7]

In my experience, patients who have undergone wrist fusion have increased function in that they are able to grasp effectively and note only some difficulty in writing on the blackboard or taking change off the counter. In patients with reasonable elbow and shoulder motion, little function is lost relative to wrist immobilization. Fusions rarely break down or need to be revised.[8] In my opinion, wrist fusion is an excellent procedure, preferable to a total wrist arthroplasty, and an operation that has provided long-term benefit to many patients with RA. This opinion is not universal[9] and convincing a patient to have a fusion rather than a total wrist arthroplasty can be difficult.

MCP Arthroplasties

Interpositional implants of silicone spacers in the MCP joints have a long history in the surgical management of RA, and there is significant controversy as to its value. The results of a survey comparing surgeons and rheumatologists regarding the value of this procedure indicated that 82% of surgeons and only 34% of the rheumatologists considered that it improved hand function.[4] Results of a multicenter trial[10] found no significant improvement in grip and pinch strength. Perhaps the wrong questions were asked. Mandl and colleagues[11] found that the highest correlation with overall satisfaction was postoperative appearance. As mentioned previously, the MCP joints operate at low pressure, and subluxations further reduce the pressure on the articular service. Destroyed MCPs are rarely, if ever, a cause of significant pain. However, patients tend to be more comfortable in relating symptoms of pain or dysfunction to their physician and often do not discuss their concerns about the appearance of their hands. This issue should be addressed in discussions regarding potential surgical interventions. There are few, if any, data on the long-term results of silicone implants, and the repaired subluxations tend to recur after several years.

However, the complication rate in MCP arthroplasties is low and removal of an infected silicone implant shares few of the morbidities experienced when an infected cemented metal prosthesis occurs in a major weight-bearing joint such as the hip. How should patients contemplating this procedure be advised? My policy has been to describe the procedure as being of low risk and primarily cosmetic with little expectation that pain or function will be greatly improved. Many patients choose to have the procedure based on this information and, more often than not, are satisfied, at least in the short term.

Procedures on the IP Joints

Surgical procedures used on the IP joints are essentially limited to fusions. The prime indication for this operation is significant joint instability with resulting dysfunction. The benefits of a fusion of an unstable IP joint of the thumb may be gratifying because of the dependence on the thumb for most critical hand functions. Because the force of leverage is geometrically proportional to the length of the lever arm, fusion of the thumb IP joint doubles the length of the lever arm and results in quadrupling the force of the pinch. The procedure, like most fusions, has few complications and is unlikely to break down with time.

REFERENCES

1. Short CL, Bauer W, Reynolds WE. Rheumatoid arthritis. Cambridge (MA): Harvard University Press; 1967.

2. Kapetanovic MC, Lindqvist E, Saxne T, et al. Orthopaedic surgery in patients with rheumatoid arthritis over 20 years: prevalence and predictive features of large joint replacement. Ann Rheum Dis 2008;67:1412–6.

3. Roberts WN, Daltroy LH, Anderson RJ. Stability of normal joint findings in persistent classical rheumatoid arthritis. Arthritis Rheum 1988;31:267–71.

4. Alderman AK, Ubel PA, Kim HM, et al. Surgical management of the rheumatoid hand: consensus and controversy among rheumatologists and hand surgeons. J Rheumatol 2003;30:1464–72.

5. Chung KC, Kotsis SV, Kim HM, et al. Reasons why rheumatoid arthritis patients seek surgical treatment for hand deformities. J Hand Surg Am 2006;31:289–94.

6. Takwale VJ, Nuttall D, Trail IA, et al. Biaxial total wrist replacement in patients with rheumatoid arthritis. Clinical review, survivorship and radiological analysis. J Bone Joint Surg Br 2002;84:622–9.

7. Radmer S, Andresen R, Sparmann M. Total wrist arthroplasty in patients with rheumatoid arthritis. J Hand Surg Am 2003;5:795–6.

8. Barbier O, Saels P, Rombouts JJ, et al. Long-term functional results of wrist arthrodesis in rheumatoid arthritis. J Hand Surg Br 1999;1:27–31.

9. Rauhaniemi J, Tiusanen H, Sipola E. Total wrist fusion: a study of 115 patients. J Hand Surg Br 2005;2:217–9.

10. Chung KC, Burns PB, Wilgis EF, et al. A multicenter clinical trial in rheumatoid arthritis comparing silicone metacarpophalangeal joint arthroplasty with medical treatment. J Hand Surg Am 2009;34(5):815–23.

11. Mandl LA, Galvin DH, Bosch JP, et al. Metacarpophalangeal arthroplasty in rheumatoid arthritis: what determines satisfaction with surgery? J Rheumatol 2002;12:2488–91.

Controversy in the Treatment of the Rheumatoid Hand: Perspective from Hand Surgery

E.F. Shaw Wilgis, MD

KEYWORDS

- Arthrodesis • Arthroplasty • Rheumatoid arthritis
- Surgery • Tendon rupture

Over the years there has been controversy between rheumatologists and surgeons regarding surgery for the correction of rheumatoid problems. There are many reasons for this controversy, and this article explores the reasons for the controversy, presents the history of rheumatoid hand surgery, and offers some possible solutions to the problem.

THE PROBLEM

Alderman and colleagues[1] conducted a study using the Healthcare Cost and Utilization Project's 1996–1997 nationwide sample to evaluate large area variations associated with the surgical management of the rheumatoid hand. This study revealed that there were varying rates of surgery and large variations in surgical practice patterns across states.[1] Many factors can contribute to this finding, including access to care and economic incentives, and a large proportion of practice variation can be explained by a disagreement among physicians regarding appropriate therapy. The discrepancy between surgeons and rheumatologists about when to intervene surgically may also contribute to this large area variation. The differences that exist in treatment philosophy may hamper effective surgical treatment of this disease for a large portion of patients with rheumatoid arthritis.

Essentially, the study confirmed that the large area variation was mainly related to differences in practice patterns between the 2 specialties, which greatly affected referral patterns. Rheumatologists tend to refer patients later in their disease, and surgeons frequently lament that patients with rheumatoid arthritis are referred too infrequently and too late.

This finding was further confirmed in another study by Alderman and colleagues[2] in which the researchers surveyed a large number of rheumatologists and surgeons across the United States and found some interesting differences of opinion. Five hundred members of the American Society for Surgery of the Hand and 500 members of the American College of Rheumatology were surveyed to understand the differences in opinions about the effectiveness of rheumatoid hand surgery. Metacarpophalangeal (MP) arthroplasty showed a remarkable difference between the specialties: among the hand surgeons who responded, 82% thought that this procedure improved hand function, whereas only 34% of the rheumatologists concurred. For small joint synovectomy and extensor tenosynovectomy, the surgeons thought that both procedures prevented tendon rupture and delayed joint destruction, whereas only 12% of rheumatologists thought that synovectomy delayed joint destruction and 54%, that it prevented tendon rupture. Regarding resection of the distal

The author did not receive any outside funding or grants in support of this work.
The Curtis National Hand Center, Union Memorial Hospital, 3333 North Calvert Street, JPB-M2, Baltimore, MD 21218, USA
E-mail address: shaw.wilgis@medstar.net

ulna, 60% to 70% of surgeons thought the procedure improved function, decreased wrist pain, prevented tendon ruptures, and increased strength. Although there was some agreement on this issue, in that 60% and 50% of rheumatologists thought that the procedure prevented tendon rupture and decreased pain, respectively, only 22% thought that it improved function and/or motion. The only area of agreement was wrist fusion. More than 90% of both groups thought that wrist fusion decreased pain, but even though 88% of surgeons thought that it improved function, only 42% of rheumatologists thought that it accomplished this goal. Similar results were found for boutonniere reconstruction. About 60% to 70% of surgeons thought that reconstruction improved hand function and aesthetic outcomes in contrast to only 24% and 63% of rheumatologists who thought that it improved function and hand aesthetic outcomes, respectively.

In summary, Alderman and colleagues[2] found that patients with rheumatoid arthritis had 2 groups of highly trained specialists caring for them, surgical and medical, but that the specialists disagree fundamentally on the effectiveness of surgery for hand deformities. Both groups agreed that surgical outcomes research for this patient population is limited. The researchers reported that there was a need for more research focused on the outcomes of surgical intervention for rheumatoid deformity followed by efforts aimed at the dissemination of the resulting data and implementation of logical treatment approaches.

There are other reasons for this discrepancy in treatment opinions. Rheumatologists treat patients on a long-term basis and review the continuum of care by determining the most pressing condition: is it the cervical spine, the hips, the elbows, the shoulders, or the hands? Surgeons, however, treat patients on an episodic basis according to the particular condition for which they are consulted. Another problem that the rheumatologist has to face is which should be considered first, the upper or the lower extremities. If patients have multiple extremities involved and need hip and possibly knee surgery for the rehabilitation of these conditions, the hands and wrists must be in fairly good function because the patient will have to walk essentially using the hands and wrists for support during the rehabilitation for the lower extremity. Conversely, if patients' hands are worse, they need to ambulate and get around with ease and without pain so they can participate in the rehabilitation of the hand. Rheumatologists face this dilemma, and often it is the joint with the most pain that gets the earliest attention.

HISTORY

The history of surgery for rheumatoid arthritis is also helpful in understanding why this dilemma exists. The treatment of rheumatoid arthritis is relatively recent. It was not until 1966 that the American College of Rheumatology devised diagnostic criteria for rheumatoid arthritis. These criteria were revised in 1987 and are now in general use.[3] The introduction of the biologic disease-modifying antirheumatic drugs has changed the medical treatment of this problem dramatically in the last 15 years.

From the history of surgery as identified by Clayton[4] in 1989, surgery for rheumatoid arthritis was started in 1943 by Smith-Petersen who advocated a radial head excision of the elbow with synovectomy and also the excision of the distal ulna and arthrodesis of the wrist. In 1948, Vaughan-Jackson described the condition of extensor tendon rupture caused by dislocated and arthritic distal ulna and recommended excision of the distal ulna with extensor tendon synovectomy.[5] There were many attempts at wrist replacement during the next 30 to 40 years, most of them resulting in failure. In the 1950s, carpal tunnel surgery, synovectomy, extensor tendon reconstruction, and wrist fusion were the main operations performed for rheumatoid arthritis. These operations were performed mainly because of ongoing pain, tendon rupture and dysfunction, and wrist pain. There were some early attempts at MP joint arthroplasty using soft tissue interposition between the metacarpals and the proximal phalanges, with realignment of the digits, mainly popularized by Vainio.[6] In 1971, Swanson[7] introduced the silicone MP joint arthroplasty (SMPA). This procedure changed the treatment of this particular condition and has withstood the passage of time. With this procedure, the MP joints are resected, cleaned of all synovium, and a silicone spacer is introduced between the metacarpals and the proximal phalanges. The extensor tendons are realigned and the wounds allowed to heal. Healing consists of the body making a fibrous capsule around the silicone implant because the implant itself is not a joint but keeps the fingers aligned while the fibrous capsule is being developed. Nevertheless, the main operations for rheumatoid arthritis continued to be extensor tendon rupture, wrist surgery, and MP joint arthroplasty of different types. Then, still in the 1970s, more extensive procedures were introduced, including realignment of the thumb by Nalebuff[8] and reconstruction of some of the smaller joints of the hand. The long-term value of any of these smaller procedures has not been proven. Most of the literature about these newer procedures report follow-up of 1 to 2 years. There is a need for studies with longer-term follow-up. In the largest series of outcomes for SMPA, Chung and colleagues[9] compared the results of surgery with medical treatment. This study examining the results of treatment of MP joint disease, which included a large group of medically treated individuals and a large group of surgically treated individuals, is ongoing. The patient groups were essentially equal in deformity. At 1 year follow-up, the surgical patients fared much better than medically treated patients in that they achieved more function, had better appearance, and had less pain. This study is being continued on a long-term basis to see how the surgical results hold up.

THE SURGICAL PERSPECTIVE

A patient who has had varying response to medical treatment after working with a rheumatologist usually on a long-term basis presents to the surgeon with problems in multiple joints and frequently, later in the disease process, with progressive deformity. The first question is "should any surgery be done?" With hip and knee reconstruction, the results are proven and successful. Also, with the cervical spine, these problems have to be dealt with so that paralysis does not ensue. However, patients with hand problems usually have learned to cope with the deformity and the gradual loss of function so that unless they complain specifically to the rheumatologist, they are unlikely to be referred for reconstructive hand surgery. Nevertheless, reconstructive hand surgery is available and hand surgeons know it is successful, at least in the short-term, especially if the patient presents before severe deformity exists.

As stated earlier in this article, the surgeon is usually faced with a single problem and only on an episodic basis, so the surgeon is looking at the particular problem for which the patient is referred, its solution, and the successful outcome.

However, when considering surgery, the surgeon must also take into account the patient's standpoint. The patient is often inadequately educated on the surgical options and the outcomes of surgery and may just have a natural aversion to the thought of surgery because of the fear of potential loss of function.

Certainly, if a rupture of extensor tendons is perfectly obvious, it will present as a much more immediate problem to the patient than the gradual decline of hand function. Some of the most worthwhile results in surgery come from arthrodesis of the wrist, excision of the distal

ulna, and arthrodesis of some of the smaller joints in the hand.

Another dilemma that the surgeon and patient face is which problem comes first and which hurts most. If patients have knee and hip pain, surgeries to correct these will probably come first, although patients probably do not realize that they must use their hands for support and will essentially have to "walk on their hands" until there is full effect of the knee and hip surgery. Once explained, the patient may choose to have reconstructive surgery of the hands and wrists before the lower extremity. The surgical plan requires intense discussion between the patient and the physician so that they can make the best choice together.

One of the main decisions that the patient and surgeon face is whether to do surgery even if the improvement is only short-lived. There are many areas in medical and surgical treatments of other conditions in which the patients have overwhelmingly chosen the short-term improvement in the quality of life.

One example of this choice is in cardiac surgery in which coronary bypass surgery and angioplasty have not been proven to prolong life over the natural progression of the disease; however, quality of life seems to be vastly improved after having these procedures. These short-term benefits have been generally accepted by patients, which explains why these procedures continue to be performed.

The same rationale can be applied to the patient facing possible surgery for rheumatoid arthritis. It is known that reconstructive surgery for thumb defects, MP joint arthroplasty, and surgery for wrist deformity result in improvement for an indefinite number of years. All medical literature on this subject report only after a 1- to 2-year follow-up. There is no question that reconstructive rheumatoid surgery needs to be evaluated on a long-term basis using comparable studies of a prospective nature. The ongoing study of MP joint arthroplasty will elucidate the answers to some of these questions.

In addition, these procedures have become far less complicated and burdensome to the patient than when they were first introduced. Most of these procedures can be performed in a short duration on an outpatient basis under a regional or local anesthetic block. Patients usually do not have to change their dosage of antirheumatoid medicines. With these improvements in surgical techniques and approach, and the fact that the procedures are smaller in scope and less intrusive to the patient, the patient's perspective about having them done may well change.

POSSIBLE SOLUTIONS

One solution to this controversy is the creation of combined treatment centers where the physician and the surgeon can see the patient together, examine and delineate the problems for the patient and then propose, together, solutions. This combined approach will be enhanced by outcome studies reporting on the long-term effect of surgical treatment. The results from hip and knee surgeries have been encouraging on a long-term basis. Although surgeries for the hand and arm have been shown to be extremely beneficial for the short-term, they have not been proven to be beneficial in the long-term.

One of the issues that must be discussed between the surgeon and the rheumatologist is whether it is right to advise correction of a problem if the results are only going to be for a short-term, for instance, only several years. This dilemma should also be discussed with the patient because the patient will ultimately make the decision. This issue has already been addressed in some specialties. For example, in coronary bypass surgery, the results have shown that although this procedure does not necessarily prolong life, the surgery makes for a better quality of life for the short-term between the operation and the ultimate outcome. Another example of a conflict occurs in the course of prostatic cancer. Extensive surgical solutions have been proposed for prostatic cancer, but there are also available medical options or there is no treatment at all, with the results being, in terms of longevity of life, about the same. However, we are interested in the quality of life.

The quality of life for a patient undergoing reconstructive hand surgery, successfully done, is definitely improved as shown by the study by Chung and colleagues,[9] at least in the short-term. It is not expected that the answers to these questions will be readily available in the near future. However, only in the combined setting, in which the disease process is regarded as a whole and the physicians and surgeons can get together to plan for the best outcome for that particular patient, will the dichotomy of thinking narrow. With the advent of combined treatment centers, the author would anticipate that the small area variations of treatment would decrease, the controversial feelings of both specialties would decrease, and the patients would benefit.

Another possible solution to the problem is education because most patients rely on their physicians for knowledge about their disease. Patients need to be better educated, and a great avenue for patient education is the Arthritis Foundation. All local chapters give out information and have meetings patients can attend. Surgeons must become part of that faculty and provide information about the various reconstructive procedures that can affect the quality of life for several years at the least.

In summary, rheumatologists do not enjoy the enthusiasm of hand surgeons for the surgical corrections of rheumatoid arthritis deformities. Surgeons know that these procedures are successful at least for some years. The long-term outcomes of these procedures need to be evaluated to provide the rheumatologist with this information. Working together, the rheumatologist and the hand surgeon should evaluate the patients to enable the patient to be adequately informed.

REFERENCES

1. Alderman AK, Chung KC, Demonner S, et al. The rheumatoid hand: a predictable disease with unpredictable surgical practice patterns. Arthritis Rheum 2002;47(5):537–42.
2. Alderman AK, Chung KC, Kim HM, et al. Effectiveness of rheumatoid hand surgery: contrasting perceptions of hand surgeons and rheumatologists. J Hand Surg Am 2003;28(1):3–11.
3. Arnett FC, Edworthy SM, Bloch DA, et al. The American Rheumatism Association 1987 revised criteria for the classification of rheumatoid arthritis. Arthritis Rheum 1988;31(3):315–24.
4. Clayton ML. Historical perspectives on surgery of the rheumatoid hand. Hand Clin 1989;5(2):111–4.
5. Vaughan-Jackson OJ. Rupture of extensor tendons by attrition at the inferior radio-ulnar joint; report of two cases. J Bone Joint Surg Br 1948;30(3):528–30.
6. Vainio K. History of surgery of rheumatoid arthritis in Europe. Scand J Rheumatol 1983;12(2):65–8.
7. Swanson AB. Flexible implant arthroplasty for arthritic finger joints: rationale, technique, and results of treatment. J Bone Joint Surg Am 1972;54(3):435–55.
8. Nalebuff EA. Present status of rheumatoid hand surgery. Am J Surg 1971;122(3):304–18.
9. Chung KC, Burns PB, Wilgis EF, et al. A multicenter clinical trial in rheumatoid arthritis comparing silicone metacarpophalangeal joint arthroplasty with medical treatment. J Hand Surg Am 2009;34(5):815–23.

Current Concepts in the Surgical Management of Rheumatoid and Osteoarthritic Hands and Wrists

Jeffrey H. Kozlow, MD, Kevin C. Chung, MD, MS*

KEYWORDS

• Rheumatoid arthritis • Osteoarthritis • Hand • Wrist

RHEUMATOID ARTHRITIS

Rheumatoid arthritis (RA) is a progressively destructive disease that affects 1% of the American population.[1] The systemic manifestations can be severe, and more than 70% of rheumatoid patients develop hand problems that are painful and disabling. Gradual loss of hand function in RA patients affects their ability for self-care and interferes with their productivity in society. The prominent hand deformity can create social stigma for RA patients (**Fig. 1**).

The RA patient presents to a surgeon searching for functional gain, pain relief, or aesthetic improvement.[2] Whether hand surgical procedures can fulfill the patient's expectations is debatable. The lack of rigorously conducted outcomes studies to support the effectiveness of hand surgery in RA patients creates persistent disagreements between hand surgeons and rheumatologists regarding the recommendations for RA hand reconstruction.[3] There are significant variations in clinical management based on gender and regional practice that further compound the issue.[4] The continuing improvement in the medical management of RA has markedly decreased the incidence of RA hand surgery. Because of the complexity of hand deformities in RA, it is important that surgeons and rheumatologists have a clear understanding of the goals and expectations of hand surgical procedures in an effort to provide a rational strategy for the overall hand rehabilitation program. In this article the authors share their extensive experience in RA hand surgery to provide a clear discussion of the indications and outcomes of its practice.

Pathophysiology

RA is a chronic, inflammatory autoimmune disease that causes joint inflammation, cartilage destruction, and ligament weakness. RA is further characterized by the formation of pannus, caused by synovial inflammation in areas of increased vascularity. The pannus invades into terminal vessels, resulting in soft tissue ischemia and stretching of adjacent, already weakened structures. Activated neutrophils from the pannus release lysosomal enzymes and free radicals destroy the articular surfaces. These destructive processes change the anatomy of the hand, leading to a gradual loss of function.

Treatment

First-line treatment of the RA hand aims to control the systemic disease. Any surgical intervention is

Supported in part by a Midcareer Investigator Award in Patient-Oriented Research (K24 AR053120) from the National Institute of Arthritis and Musculoskeletal and Skin Diseases (to Dr Kevin C. Chung).
Section of Plastic Surgery, Department of Surgery, University of Michigan Medical School, 2130 Taubman Center, SPC 5340, 1500 East Medical Center Drive, Ann Arbor, MI 48109-0340, USA
* Corresponding author.
E-mail address: kecchung@umich.edu

Hand Clin 27 (2011) 31–41
doi:10.1016/j.hcl.2010.09.003
0749-0712/11/$ — see front matter. Published by Elsevier Inc.

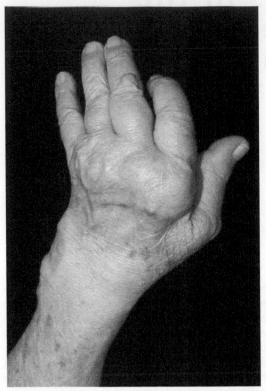

Fig. 1. A severely deformed rheumatoid hand including: (1) extensor tenosynovitis over the MCP joints, (2) ulnar deviation of the digits, (3) boutonniere deformity of the thumb, and (4) collapse of the carpus.

futile without controlling the systemic inflammation, as surgical repairs cannot withstand the inflammatory challenge of uncontrolled disease. Hand surgeons must work closely with rheumatologists when contemplating surgical treatment. Anti-inflammatory medications are weaned as tolerated to decrease the risk of wound-healing complications. Working closely with certified hand therapists in the pre- and postoperative periods is necessary to ensure the best outcomes. The first step in any planned surgical intervention is early evaluation by a hand surgeon experienced with RA to develop a treatment program that minimizes the incidence of uncorrectable late deformities.

RA hand surgery is divided into prophylactic and reconstructive procedures. Prophylactic procedures include tenosynovectomy, joint synovectomy, and tendon rebalancing. These prophylactic procedures may delay the destructive RA processes, extending the useful life span of tendons and joints. Reconstructive procedures are often more complex than prophylactic procedures. Reconstructive procedures include arthrodesis,

arthroplasty, and tendon transfer. The surgical treatment algorithm depends on the individual patient, the involved joints, and the desired outcome. Regardless of the operative procedure, the surgeon must discuss the limitations and risks of surgery with the patient to avoid unrealistic postoperative expectations. RA hand surgery never restores normal function.

Preoperative evaluation

During the initial consultation, the surgeon should understand the patient's concerns regarding hand function and hand appearance. Deformity alone is not an indication for proposing surgical treatment. Rather, the surgeon ought to assess the patient's hand impairment in work and daily activities to render recommendations as to whether surgical treatment can be beneficial. Many RA patients can adapt to their hand deformities over time. The challenge for the hand surgeon is to evaluate whether the surgical intervention can enhance patient function. The surgeon should have sufficient prescience to recommend procedures that may prevent the development of future deformities. Some patients may also be concerned about the appearance of the deformed hand. Enhancing the appearance of an RA hand may have unrecognized benefit to the patients' self-esteem.

An experienced RA surgeon will consider the priority of reconstruction. For example, patients should undergo lower extremity procedures first to avoid the stress from crutches or walker on the reconstructed upper limbs. In addition, proximal joints should be reconstructed before distal joints. A destroyed elbow will hamper wrist and hand function. The elbow should be treated first, followed by the wrist and the hand. Because radial deviation of the wrist will cause ulnar subluxation of the metacarpophalangeal (MCP) joints, wrist deformity is corrected before undertaking MCP joint reconstruction.

Three-view radiographs of the hands and wrists are mandatory to evaluate radiographic changes in the joints. The amount of articular or bony destruction seen on radiographs does not necessarily correlate with patients' complaints. Often, patients with minimal wrist pain have advanced wrist collapse on radiographs. Preoperative evaluation of the neck and cervical spine is essential because a substantial proportion of RA patients have atlantoaxial subluxation. Instability of the cervical spine should be evaluated before undergoing surgical procedures. Ideally, regional anesthesia is preferred, but some patients may require general anesthesia.

Prophylactic procedures

Prophylactic surgical procedures in the rheumatoid patient include tenosynovectomy, joint synovectomy, and tendon rebalancing. Tenosynovectomy is the surgical removal of inflamed synovial tissues surrounding a tendon, whereas joint synovectomy is the removal of inflamed synovial tissue within a joint. Excision of inflamed synovial tissue is ideally performed prior to irreversible joint destruction. Removing inflamed and hypertrophic peritendinous synovial tissues can enhance tendon gliding and improve finger motion. Excising bulging synovial tissues from joints should decrease pain. Because tendons and ligaments around joints may be stretched from hypertrophic synovium, tendon rebalancing can restored the anatomic positions of the displaced tendons and ligaments.

Tenosynovectomy Inflammation of the synovial lining of extensor tendons leads to swelling over the dorsal hand and wrist. These synovial tissues can invade the tendons and cause them to rupture. Extensor tenosynovectomy is recommended when synovitis persists for 3 to 6 months despite aggressive medical management. Extensor tendon rupture should be differentiated from other causes of extension lag including: (1) extensor tendon subluxation at the MCP joints, (2) MCP joint dislocations, and (3) posterior interosseous nerve (PIN) palsy. When the extensor tendon is subluxed between the head of the metacarpals, it acts as an MCP joint flexor instead of an extensor. The

course of the extensor tendons is seen ulnar to the head of the metacarpals. When the fingers are extended passively, the subluxed extensor tendons can maintain partial finger extension. Joint subluxation is marked by prominent metacarpal heads and the proximal phalanges resting volar to the metacarpals. Radiographs will confirm the subluxation. Inability to extend any of the digits or thumb suggests a PIN injury attributable to inflammation around the nerve at the radiohumeral joint.

A dorsal longitudinal incision is used for extensor tenosynovectomy to expose all extensor compartments. Following tenosynovectomy, the extensor retinaculum can be split in half transversely. One half is place under the tendons to shield the extensor tendons from the eroded wrist bones and the other half is placed over the tendons to prevent bowstringing. **Fig. 2** demonstrates an example of extensor tenosynovectomy. The terminal branch of the PIN, which rests on the floor of the fourth extensor compartment, can be excised to denervate the wrist joint if there is associated wrist pain.

At the MCP joints, a tendon rebalancing procedure is often combined with MCP joint synovectomy. The stretched radial sagittal band is opened to provide access to the joint for synovectomy. The radial sagittal band is then imbricated to relocate the extensor tendons. The deforming ulnar lateral band can be divided distally from the index, middle, and ring fingers to transfer to the extensor tendons of the middle, ring, and little fingers to maintain the extensor tendon

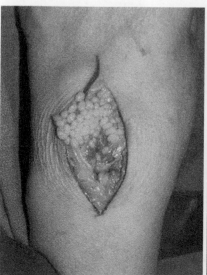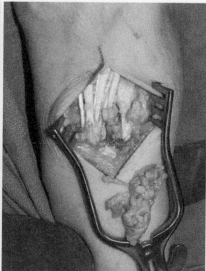

Fig. 2. Intraoperative photographs demonstrating extensor tenosynovitis with rice bodies (*left*), and subsequent removal of the extensor tenosinovium (*right*).

in the central position. This intrinsic transfer procedure is used when the MCP joint is still passively reducible by transferring the tight ulnar intrinsic tendons to bring the fingers back into alignment. The abductor quinti minimi should be released because it is often tight and draws the little finger ulnarly. The index finger is realigned by tightening the radial sagittal band, as there is no adjacent finger to provide the ulnar lateral band. Radial deviation of the wrist can contribute to ulnar deviation of the fingers. Transferring the extensor carpi radialis longus (ECRL) tendon, which inserts over the index metacarpal, to the extensor carpi ulnaris (ECU) can balance the wrist. Not only can this transfer remove the deforming radial force on the wrist, the ECRL transfer can elevate the often volarly subluxed ECU tendon and provide a more ulnar, dorsal pull to the wrist.

The flexor system can also be affected by synovitis. The increased bulk in the flexor tendon sheath causes less active flexion than passive flexion of the fingers. The joints in the fingers are still mobile and can be passively flexed, but the inflamed flexor tendons are not able to pull the fingers actively into flexion. In addition, sufficient synovial tissue buildup in the flexor tendons can cause triggering of the fingers at either the A1 pulley or the carpal tunnel. Unlike the traditional "trigger finger," whereby release of the A1 pulley is the preferred treatment, in RA trigger it is recommended that the A1 pulley is preserved to support the MCP joints from ulnar deviating forces. The preferred method is removal of the synovial tissue and excision of a slip of the flexor digitorum superficialis (FDS) tendon to decrease the volume within the pulley system (**Fig. 3**). Carpal tunnel release treats the wrist trigger and alleviates median nerve compression.

Joint synovectomy Intra-articular inflammation of the wrist, MCP, or proximal interphalangeal (PIP) joints causes pain and decreases motion. Synovitis leads to laxity of the joint capsule, collateral ligaments, and volar plate. The continued stretching of the support ligaments results in tendon imbalances. The rationale for early joint synovectomy is to remove the diseased synovium prior to articular cartilage destruction and supporting ligament attenuation. For MCP joint synovitis, 6 to 9 months of medical management is recommended before considering surgery. Persistent, localized joint synovitis may benefit from synovectomy, but the long-term benefit of surgery in ameliorating joint destruction has not been shown in well-conducted trials.

The surgeon should discuss with the patient preoperatively that these are prophylactic and not curative procedures. While the literature suggests synovectomy does provide some palliation of symptoms, the outcomes data on the effectiveness of these procedures are still limited. Perceptions of the success rate of these procedures differ

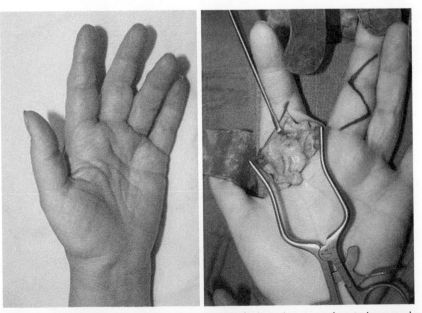

Fig. 3. A patient presenting with flexor tenosynovitis and digital triggering secondary to increased mass at the A1 pulley (*left*) along with the corresponding intraoperative photograph (*right*).

between rheumatologists and hand surgeons.[5] The introduction of new RA medications has been quite effective in treating synovitis and the rate of synovectomy procedures is decreasing.

Reconstructive procedures

Wrist The wrist is the earliest and most frequent site of RA hand disease. Destruction of the ulnar carpal ligamentous structures leads to a syndrome called caput ulna syndrome. This "ulnar head syndrome" is marked by dorsal subluxation of the distal ulna. The inflammation of the dorsal soft tissue envelope leads to weakening of the dorsal supporting structures. Supination of the carpus subsequently occurs as a result of loss of dorsal support and the volar displacing force of the flexor tendons. This volarly displacing force is exacerbated by volar subluxation of the ECU. Inflammation of the radial sided structures further deforms the wrist. Unopposed pull of the radial wrist extensors leads to radial deviation of the metacarpals and a resultant ulnar deviation of the phalanges. In addition, the loss of dorsal soft tissue support leads to dorsal dislocation of the ulnar head and weakening of the distal radial-ulnar joint (DRUJ). In advanced disease, there is complete collapse of the wrist with volar

dislocation of the carpus and dissociation of the DRUJ. Radiographs are often worse than the clinical picture. Treatment is targeted at patient concerns and not radiographic findings. Operative interventions for the RA wrist are mainly reconstructive. Total synovectomy is impossible because access to the many recesses in the wrist joint is difficult and partial synovectomy alone provides limited long-term benefit.

The wrist is a complex joint, and surgical interventions need to address the DRUJ, radiocarpal joint, and midcarpal joint. For moderate disease in a patient with limited functional demand distal ulna resection, or Darrach procedure, is beneficial. An incision is made over the distal ulna to expose the sixth compartment. The sheath over the distal ulna is incised and an oblique osteotomy is made over the neck of the ulna head (**Fig. 4**). Synovectomy of the DRUJ and relocation of the ECU are performed concurrently. Alternatively, ECRL can be transferred to the ECU to improve alignment. The forearm is now supinated to seat the distal ulna stump volarly. The dorsal capsule is closed tightly over the distal ulna stump. This procedure is not advised when the wrist is unstable because the lack of ulna head support may lead to ulnar subluxation of the carpus. In these cases, the

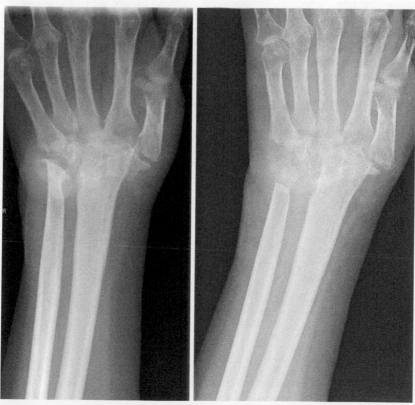

Fig. 4. Severe ulnar head destruction (*left*) is treated by distal ulnar resection (*right*).

Suave-Kapandji procedure is preferred. Instead of resection of the distal ulna, a segmental resection is performed proximally. The distal ulnar remnant is then fused to the sigmoid notch of the distal radius. Arthrodesis is performed using either K-wires or an interfragment screw.

Radiocarpal articular wear requires arthroplasty or arthrodesis (**Fig. 5**). Both procedures are indicated for deformity and instability that interfere with function or cause persistent pain. Prerequisite requirements for arthroplasty include good preoperative wrist motion, functional wrist tendons, and good bone stock. In addition, adequate soft tissue is necessary to stabilize the wrist implant. Wrist arthroplasty is a predictable procedure and has a low complication rate. It is contraindicated in patients with severe shoulder and elbow diseases because patients may not be able to adapt to loss of motion in all 3 joints. Compared with arthrodesis, the postoperative rehabilitation program for arthroplasty is generally more difficult and is associated with a higher risk of complications. The wrist mobility with arthroplasty is traded for the predictability with arthrodesis. Older methods of arthroplasty included the use of silicone or metal/polyethylene implants. An expanding number of total wrist replacement systems are increasing reconstructive options.[6] Complications of wrist arthroplasty include fracture, infection, implant failure, implant dislocation, and implant loosening. For patients with a bilateral wrist problem, arthrodesis is recommended in the dominant hand to maintain stability for gripping and power. The nondominant hand is treated with arthroplasty to maintain some joint motion needed for self-hygiene. Destruction of the radiocarpal joint with preservation of the midcarpal joint may be treated with limited arthrodesis, which maintains about 25% to 50% of wrist motion through motion at the midcarpal joint.

Metacarpophalangeal joint The MCP joint is the key joint for finger function. When one grips an object, the arc of motion is initiated at the MCP joint, then the PIP and distal interphalangeal (DIP) joints. Therefore, motion at the MCP joints of the fingers must be maintained for adequate hand function. The cam design of the MCP joint is stable in flexion during grip because of tightening of the collateral ligaments, but is mobile in extension to manipulate objects. The typical ulnar deviation of the MCP joints is postulated to result from the following causes. First, the flexor and extensor tendons approach the MCP joints over the ulnar sides, leading to a natural tendency for ulnar deviation with extension. Second, the normal pinch forces further direct the phalanges ulnarly. Third, radial deviation of the wrist and metacarpals in the RA hand combined with radial sagittal band attenuation leads to further ulnar shifting of the extensor tendons. These factors contribute to gradual tightening of the ulnar intrinsic tendons, resulting in ulnar and volar subluxation at the MCP joints.

The RA patient with minimal pain and good hand function is best treated without an operation. When synovectomy is not applicable due to joint destruction, MCP arthroplasty should be considered. Traditional arthroplasty is performed with a silicone implant (**Fig. 6**). After removing the diseased joints, the silicone spacer implant is inserted. The silicone implants are easy to place

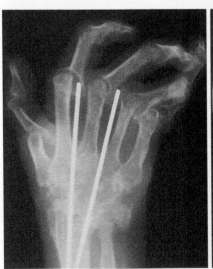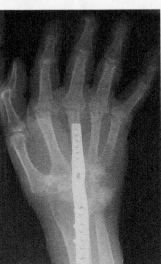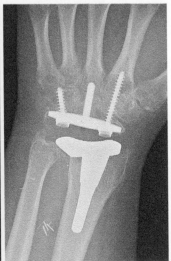

Fig. 5. Surgical treatment options of the rheumatoid wrist includes arthrodesis using Steinmann pins (*left*) or plating (*center*). Alternatively, prosthetic total wrist arthroplasty (*right*) can be performed.

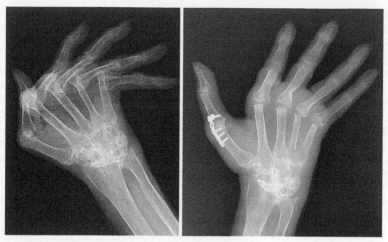

Fig. 6. Preoperative radiographs demonstrating MCP disease with joint destruction and subluxation (*left*). Following Swanson arthroplasty and realignment procedures, the hand is closer to a normal posture (*right*).

but fracture of the implants are not uncommon. The crucial part of the operation is to centralize the extensor tendons by stabilizing the radial ligament support. One must correct radial wrist deformity before MCP arthroplasty to avoid persistent ulnar forces on the reconstructed MCP joints. Following MCP arthroplasty, patients report significant improvement in function, aesthetic appearance, and overall satisfaction.[7]

Interphalangeal joints Digital deformities in the rheumatoid hand are either swan-neck or boutonniere deformities. Swan-neck deformity is defined by hyperextension of the PIP and flexion of the DIP joint (**Fig. 7**). The functional consequence of a swan-neck deformity is an inability to grasp objects because of hyperextension of the PIP joint. There are 4 initiating causes for a swan-neck deformity. First, extensor rupture at the terminal insertion creates a mallet finger that can progress to hyperextension of the PIP joint as the extensor tendon migrates proximally to increase the extensor force over the PIP joint. Second, PIP synovitis leads to volar plate laxity.

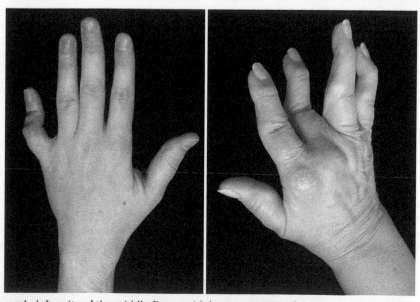

Fig. 7. A swan-neck deformity of the middle finger with hyperextension of the PIP and flexion of the DIP is shown on the left. For comparison, a boutonniere deformity of the small finger with flexion of the PIP and hyperextension of the DIP is shown on the right.

Third, FDS tendon rupture at its insertion at the PIP joint leads to increased extensor force at the PIP joint. Lastly, intrinsic tendon tightness from MCP joint dislocation hyperextends the PIP joint. Initially, the deformity is correctable and soft tissue reconstruction may correct the deformity. Over time the deformity may become fixed, and secondary joint contracture and articular wear may require joint procedures such as arthroplasty or arthrodesis.

To determine treatment for flexible swan-neck deformity, one should understand the etiology of the deformity. For example, if the deformity is caused by intrinsic tendon tightness and MCP joint subluxation, cross-intrinsic transfer (for mild subluxation) or resection arthroplasty will correct the problem. If the problem is at the PIP joint, providing more flexion force to the PIP joint can be helpful. For example, a slip of the FDS tendon can be divided proximally and sutured to the A1 pulley or to the metacarpal to prevent hyperextension of the PIP joint. Alternatively, the ulnar slip of the lateral band can be detached proximally and rerouted volar to the Cleland ligament so that it is now volar to the axis of the PIP joint. By securing the lateral band to the bone, hyperextension is prevented and the deformity is corrected. If the problem arises from the DIP joint, then DIP joint fusion is the most predictable procedure.

The boutonniere (or button-hole) deformity has only one cause, which is rupture of the central extensor tendon over the PIP joint. The head of the proximal phalanx can "button-hole" through the ruptured extensor tendon. In this deformity, the MCP joint is hyperextended, the PIP joint is flexed, and the DIP joint is hyperextended (see **Fig. 7**). The hypertrophic synovium at the PIP joint stretches the central extensor tendon. Secondary changes include volar displacement of the lateral bands and tightening of the oblique retinacular ligament, which hyperextend the DIP joint. Compensatory MCP hyperextension occurs because the patient tries to extend the fingers to get around objects. Early synovectomy may prevent the secondary changes. When secondary changes occur and the joint can still be reduced, terminal tenotomy will increase the tension over the PIP joint and correct the deformity. The DIP joint can still extend via the oblique retinacular ligament. If the joint is destroyed, the choices are limited to arthroplasty or arthrodesis.

Patients with boutonniere deformity can often compensate for the deformity. Power grip is retained due to the flexion deformity at the PIP joint. Surgical correction may rob the patient of the ability to fully flex the PIP joints, resulting in loss of power grip in the ulnar digits. Therefore, the decision to proceed with surgery on an ulnar-sided boutonniere deformity must be considered carefully. Boutonniere deformity is exceedingly difficult to treat. Although the deformity is unsightly, patients can often adapt. In contrast, swan-neck deformity is easier to treat because patients often have an inability to grasp objects due to the extension posture at the PIP joints. Thus, the outcomes after treating a swan-neck deformity are better than for boutonniere deformity.

Thumb Thumb deformities in the rheumatoid hand can be considered as boutonniere or swan-neck deformities, although the thumb having 2 phalanges is different from the fingers. In thumb boutonniere deformity, the MCP joint is flexed and the IP joint hyperextended. Thumb boutonniere deformity occurs from MCP joint synovitis, leading to attenuation of extensor pollicis brevis (EPB), which inserts at the proximal phalanx. Similarly, the distension of the MCP joint stretches the extensor hood and causes volar subluxation of the extensor pollicis longus (EPL) tendon, which now flexes the MCP joint. For passively correctable disease, the treatment is synovectomy and rerouting of the EPL to extend the MCP joint. If the MCP joint deformity becomes fixed, MCP arthrodesis should be performed if the carpometacarpal (CMC) and IP joints are functional.

In swan-neck deformities, the deformity starts at the CMC joint. Radial and dorsal subluxation of the CMC joints results in an adduction contracture of the metacarpal. Compensatory MCP joint hyperextension occurs. CMC arthroplasty and volar tenodesis of the MCP joint (to correct for the compensatory MCP joint hyperextension) is recommended unless damage to the MCP joint is severe. In these cases, MCP arthrodesis is performed.

Tendon rupture Medical and surgical management of tenosynovitis can prevent tendon rupture. Unfortunately, many RA patients do not present to a hand surgeon until tendon rupture has already occurred. An examination of a patient with extensor tendon lag should be able to differentiate between tendon rupture and other causes such as MCP joint subluxation or extensor tendon dislocation. The junctura between extensor tendons may still extend the ring or little fingers if the rupture is proximal, but the patient may lack the final 10° to 20° of MCP joint extension. In planning reconstruction, one should also treat the underlying causes of extensor tendon rupture by removing the infiltrating synovial tissues or by excising a prominent arthritic distal ulna. For ruptured flexor tendons, one should debride the volarly-subluxed distal scaphoid. When performing tenosynovectomy, the surgeon should always consider the possibility of finding ruptured tendons encased by the synovial tissues. The patient should be informed that tendon reconstructive procedures may be necessary as part of the synovectomy.

Tendon ruptures can be reconstructed by primary repair, tendon transfer, or tendon grafting. For a single tendon rupture that is detected early, it is theoretically possible to perform primary repair. However, the tendon quality is generally poor because the ends of the tendon are frayed from inflammation and attrition. Extensor tendon ruptures occur in the little finger first and then progress radially (**Fig. 8**). The Vaughn-Jackson syndrome refers to the little finger extensor tendon rupture from a prominent, eroded distal ulna. Both the extensor digitorum communis (EDC) and extensor digiti minimi of the little finger must rupture to develop an extension lag. It is often difficult to detect the rupture because the onset may be insidious and patients may still able to extend the little finger through the junctura attachment to the ring finger. When the little finger extensor is ruptured, the distal end can be attached to the ring finger. For ruptures of the ring and little fingers, attachment of the little finger extensor tendon to the intact middle finger will cause excessive ulnar deviation of the little finger. The senior author's preference is to transfer the extensor indicis proprius (EIP) tendon to power both the ring and little fingers. For ruptures of middle, ring, and little fingers, the

middle finger can be attached to the EDC of the index while the EIP can power the ring and little fingers. For rupture of all 4 finger extensor tendons, which is uncommon and is an unacceptable neglect by the patient and the physician, one can use the FDS tendons for the middle and ring fingers to power the extensors.

On the flexor side, the most common tendon to rupture is the flexor pollicis longus (FPL) from abrasion over the volarly-displaced scaphoid. This lesion is also known as the Mannerfelt lesion. FPL rupture may be overlooked because it tends to occur in an already nonfunctional thumb. Tendon grafting is used to repair FPL if the rupture is detected within 4 to 6 weeks before myostatic contracture of the FPL muscle hinders recovery of muscle function. In late presentation, brachioradialis or FDS of the index finger are ready donors for transfer to the FPL.

Summary

The care of the rheumatoid patient is complex and challenging. One should always ask the patient about his or her needs when planning reconstruction. Deformity is not an indication for reconstruction because patients can often compensate for their deformity. Rheumatologists must also be engaged in the discussion about reconstruction, and can be particularly helpful in pre- and postoperative management of patients' medications. A well-informed patient as regards outcomes and complications is a patient who will derive the maximum benefit from a well-conceived surgical treatment program.[8]

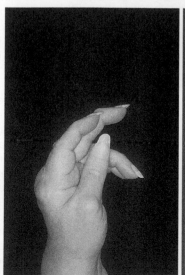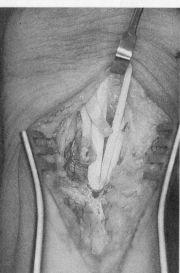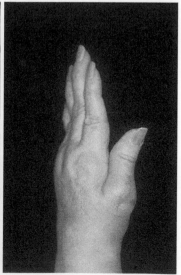

Fig. 8. This patient initially presented with loss of small and ring finger extension (*left*). Tendon rupture was found intraoperatively (*middle*). Following tendon transfer, the patient regained full extension.

OSTEOARTHRITIS

Osteoarthritis (OA) of the hand clinically affects 3% to 7% of adults.[9] Elderly women are more likely to have hand involvement as compared with men. The CMC joint of the thumb and the IP joints of the digits are most frequently affected. OA is characterized by degradation of cartilage, resulting in joint destruction and osteophyte formation (**Fig. 9**). There appears to be a genetic component to OA in the development of hand disease. The underlying etiology is repetitive trauma inducing local chondrocytes to release degradative enzymes that damage the cartilage. In contrast to RA, OA has less inflammatory reaction in the joints. The initial treatment of OA is medication and therapy. Steroid injection into affected joints can provide short-term relief. Repeat injections, however, carry a cumulative risk of weakening the soft tissue and may cause thinning and hypopigmentation of the skin.

Treatment

Preoperative evaluation
Patients with OA may exhibit classic Heberden and Bouchard nodes located at the DIP and PIP joints, respectively. Early radiographic findings include joint space narrowing and presence of osteophytes. Subchondral cyst and sclerosis are signs of more advanced disease. Symptom severity does not always correlate with radiographic findings; therefore, interventions should be based on patients' complaints. A full medical workup is necessary before surgery given the multiple comorbidities often seen in the typical elderly OA patient.

Operative procedures
Thumb carpometacarpal joint OA in the trapeziometacarpal joint is particularly common in perimenopausal women. Patients often complain of thumb weakness because of pain. Examination may reveal a positive grind test, which is axial compression of the joint causing pain from the denuded articular surfaces rubbing against each other. The initial treatment may consist of splinting or steroid injection into the joint. Early disease may require tendon reconstruction of the volar beak ligament using a strip of flexor carpi radialis (FCR) tendon. A metacarpal osteotomy that redistributes force to the dorsal portion of the joint may stabilize the joint and decrease abnormal wear patterns. However, most patients presenting to surgeons already have sufficient joint destruction that requires a more complex reconstructive approach.

For degenerative changes in the thumb CMC joint, surgical treatment is based on trapeziectomy

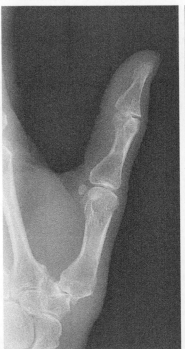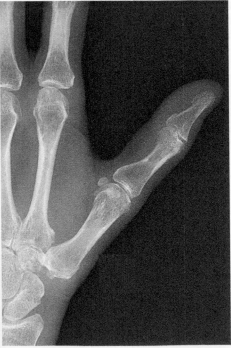

Fig. 9. These radiographs highlight the OA thumb with CMC destruction (*left*) and the subsequent postoperative radiograph following trapeziectomy and ligament reconstruction (*right*).

augmented by adjuvant procedures including ligament reconstruction and tendon interposition (LRTI), abductor pollicis longus suspensionplasty, trapeziometacarpal joint replacement, or CMC arthrodesis (see **Fig. 9**). The LRTI procedure involves resection of the trapezium with insertion of the FCR tendon through the base of the thumb metacarpal to stabilize the base of the thumb. The void created by the trapeziectomy is filled with the remaining FCR tendon. The abductor pollicis longus (APL) suspensionplasty uses the dorsal slip of the APL by weaving the tendon into the ECRL. This procedure is the current preferred technique by the senior author. Data comparing outcomes amongst the various procedures are limited and inconclusive. A recent systematic review showed that no one procedure is significantly better. It appears that trapeziectomy alone has the lowest complication rate and that trapeziectomy with LRTI has the highest complication rate.[10]

For heavy laborers, trapeziometacarpal fusion is a reasonable option. Arthrodesis with 30° to 40° of abduction, 15° to 20° of extension, and sufficient pronation to allow tip-to-tip pinch function produces the best functional outcome. A common pitfall in treating thumb CMC disease is the failure to treat concomitant hyperextension of the MCP joint. The untreated compensatory hyperextension of the thumb MCP puts stress on the reconstructed CMC joint and causes failure of this procedure. Volar capsulodesis by advancing the volar plate proximally or MCP fusion are common ancillary procedures.

Interphalangeal joints Treatment of the PIP joint in an OA hand is dependent on location. In general, the radial digits tend to be treated with arthrodesis to provide a strong post for pinch. By contrast, the ulnar digits require motion and should undergo arthroplasty. The method of arthrodesis is dependent on personal experience. Options include K-wires, screws, or tension banding. Silicone arthroplasty gives limited motion of 30° to 40° at the PIP joints, and lateral instability is common. Recent advances in pyrolytic carbon implants has led to greater motion, but complications such as dislocation of the implant can be particularly difficult to treat. When considering fusion, the PIP joint of the index finger is fused at 25° of flexion, advancing by 5° for each finger ulnarly.

The DIP joint is also commonly affected in OA. Enlarged osteophytes can be removed, and when the joint is destroyed, fusion is an excellent option. Arthroplasty is not indicated because the DIP joints require stability. Fusion at about 5° to 10° of flexion is appropriate.

SUMMARY

The hand manifestations of OA can be debilitating. The initial treatment is still medical, and many patients can do well with splinting and hand therapy. Appropriate use of arthroplasty and arthrodesis for the affected joints requires careful consideration of the patient's needs for the affected digits.

REFERENCES

1. Lawrence RC, Helmick CG, Arnett FC, et al. Estimates of the prevalence of arthritis and selected musculoskeletal disorders in the United States. Arthritis Rheum 1998;41:778–99.
2. Chung KC, Kotsis SV, Kim HM, et al. Reasons why rheumatoid arthritis patients seek surgical treatment for hand deformities. J Hand Surg Am 2006;31:289–94.
3. Ghattas L, Mascella F, Pomponio G. Hand surgery in rheumatoid arthritis: state of the art and suggestions for research. Rheumatology 2005;44:834–45.
4. Alderman AK, Chung KC, Demonner S, et al. The rheumatoid hand: a predictable disease with unpredictable surgical practice patterns. Arthritis Rheum 2005;47:537–42.
5. Alderman AK, Chung KC, Kim HM, et al. Effectiveness of rheumatoid hand surgery: contrasting perceptions of hand surgeons and rheumatologists. J Hand Surg Am 2003;28:3–11.
6. Papp SR, Athwal GS, Pichora DR. The rheumatoid wrist. J Am Acad Orthop Surg 2006;14:65–77.
7. Chung KC, Kotsis SV, Kim HM. A prospective outcomes study of Swanson metacarpophalangeal joint arthroplasty for the rheumatoid hand. J Hand Surg Am 2004;29:646–53.
8. Souter W. Planning treatment of the rheumatoid hand. Hand 1979;11:3–15.
9. Fumagalli M, Pieracarlo SP, Atzent F. Hand osteoarthritis. Semin Arthritis Rheum 2005;34(6 Suppl 2): 47–52.
10. Wajon A, Ada L, Edmunds I. Surgery for the thumb (trapeziometacarpal joint) osteoarthritis. Cochrane Database Syst Rev 2005;(4):1–61.

Rheumatoid Elbow

George S.M. Dyer, MD[a,b],*, Philip E. Blazar, MD[a]

KEYWORDS

- Rheumatoid arthritis • Elbow • Elbow degeneration
- Total elbow arthroplasty

The elbow is often involved in the progression of rheumatoid arthritis (RA).[1] Because of the elbow's unique role in maneuvering and positioning the hand in space, loss of normal elbow motion, loss of stability, or increased pain with the use of the elbow are all significant sources of impairment in patients with rheumatoid arthritis. The improvements in disease-modifying medications have greatly diminished the prevalence of severe elbow degeneration among patients with rheumatoid arthritis. However, it has not eliminated it. Abe and colleagues[2] followed disease activity in the course of elbow degeneration in 118 elbows in 59 subjects who began treatment using modern antirheumatic drugs over a 10-year period. At 10 years, 30 of 120 progressed to Larsen grade 3 changes despite medication.

Surgery remains necessary for many patients whose disease involves the elbow. Surgical management varies according to the age of patients and the stage of the disease. The goal of early intervention is to minimize or delay the loss of articular and ligamentous anatomy. In later stages, excising or creating interposition for arthritic joint surfaces may delay the need for prosthetic replacement. Once the joint is significantly destroyed, arthroplasty is the remaining option. Although results of total elbow arthroplasty are comparable in patients with rheumatoid arthritis to those in other patients, there are particular concerns for this surgery.

ELBOW ANATOMY

The elbow is uniquely and marvelously adapted for its role positioning the hand in space. It comprises 2 articulations. The ulno-humeral joint permits function and extension over nearly a 180° arc, with a stable rigid endpoint at full extension. The radiocapitellar joint and proximal radioulnar joints permit an independent 180° arc of rotation of the forearm unit in all positions of elbow flexion. Neither of these bony articulations has much intrinsic stability. Stability to varus and valgus stress is conferred by the radial and ulnar lateral collateral ligaments. Rotational stability is conferred by the annular ligament and by the elbow joint capsule.

PATHOPHYSIOLOGY OF RA IN THE ELBOW

Rheumatoid arthritis is fundamentally an inflammatory disease of soft tissue. The bony abnormalities and cartilage loss are secondary effects, resulting from the erosive properties of the inflammatory pannus. It is helpful to bear this in mind when approaching patients with rheumatoid with elbow involvement.

At the early stages of disease, stopping or modifying the inflammatory process will arrest advancement of bony changes. If stopping or modifying the inflammatory process fails, physical removal of the inflammatory pannus (synovectomy) may significantly forestall further articular degeneration. Only after the failure of these interventions is joint replacement normally considered.

Inflammatory changes also affect the ligaments around the elbow joint. Instability may be a dominant feature of presentation in the elbow. Failure to address elbow stability may affect the outcome of other interventions.

CLINICAL PRESENTATION

The clinical approach to patients with rheumatoid arthritis affecting the elbow requires particular care. Several staging systems have been developed

[a] VA Boston Healthcare, 150 South Huntington Avenue, Jamaica Plain, MA 02130, USA
[b] Hand/Upper Extremity Service, Department of Orthopaedic Surgery, Brigham and Women's Hospital, Harvard Medical School, 75 Francis Street, Boston, MA 02115, USA
* Corresponding author. Hand/Upper Extremity Service, Department of Orthopaedic Surgery, Brigham and Women's Hospital, Harvard Medical School, 75 Francis Street, Boston, MA 02115.
E-mail address: GDYER@PARTNERS.ORG

Hand Clin 27 (2011) 43–48
doi:10.1016/j.hcl.2010.10.003
0749-0712/11/$ — see front matter © 2011 Elsevier Inc. All rights reserved.

and these generally include both radiographic criteria and clinical symptoms. Rheumatoid disease of the elbow rarely occurs in isolation. Account must be taken of impairments at the hands and wrists distally, as well as at the shoulder proximally. In general, patients with advanced rheumatoid arthritis are both remarkably adaptable, adjusting functionally to their impairments, and also particularly able to share in the decision-making about management of their disease.

For purposes of research and to adopt a common frame of reference to describe radiographic changes, the Larsen grading system is often used. This grading system ranges from Grade 0 (no change); Grade II (showing periarticular erosions with some joint-space narrowing); Grade III (with moderate joint destruction); Grade IV (having severe destruction, collapse, and significant periarticular erosions); and Grade V (grossly mutilating changes).

However, severity of radiograph changes is never the only indication for surgical intervention. One useful classification system is the Mayo classification, which is a combination of clinical symptoms and radiograph assessment. Mayo grades I and II are marked predominantly by synovitis. Grade II is defined by clinical symptoms that cannot be controlled by medication alone. Mayo grades III and IV are marked by increasing degrees of joint destruction, and synovitis may be less apparent or quiescent.

MANAGEMENT

Clearly the first stage of management is to maximize medical therapy. Modern disease modifying agents have truly revolutionized the management of this disease. It is therefore assumed that the subsequent discussion concerns patients in whom these nonsurgical options have failed.

Intraarticular Injection

Intraarticular injection of corticosteroid may be helpful in early stages. Variable precision has been reported in injections performed blindly in an office setting; however, follow-up studies demonstrate equal effectiveness of ultrasound-guided injection.[3] Intraarticular injection of modern disease-modifying medication, such as etanercept, has been tried with disappointing results that are no better than corticosteroid.[4]

Synovectomy and Radial Head Excision

If the medical control of inflammatory synovitis fails, it may be physically removed through surgical synovectomy. This procedure is generally performed through a lateral approach, and if sufficiently deformed by disease involvement, the radial head may be excised at the same time. Particular care must be taken to perform as thorough a synovectomy as possible. It may be difficult to reach the medial and posterior aspects of the elbow through a lateral approach.

Fuerst and colleagues[5] presented a carefully performed follow-up of open synovectomy. They separated early synovectomy (performed with radiographic changes of Larsen grades I and II and preserving the radial head) from late synovectomy (performed with Larsen grades III and IV) and performed together with radial head excision. For early synovectomy they reported a survival rate (no further operations) of 91% at 5 years and 78% at 10 years. For late synovectomy they reported a survival rate of 82% at 5 years and 66% at 10 years.

Long-term follow-up of open synovectomy, with or without excision of the radial head, shows durable improvements in pain motion and daily functioning in many patients.[6]

ROLE OF ARTHROSCOPY

There has been considerable interest in performing synovectomy with the use of an arthroscope rather than through an open incision. In addition to the obvious advantages of less exposure and smaller incisions, it may be possible to reach the less accessible aspects of the elbow through an approach with multiple portals rather than with a single lateral incision.

Nemoto and colleagues[7] (2004) reported on arthroscopic synovectomy without resection of the radial head with a short follow-up of 37 months. There were significant and stable results over that period. Horiuchi and colleagues[8] reported on arthroscopic synovectomy in 29 elbows. They found good short-term relief of pain and improvement in Mayo score but a high rate of progression to total elbow replacement in subjects with higher-grade changes at the time of synovectomy.

In a nonrandomized trial, Tanaka and colleagues[9] compared results of open versus arthroscopic synovectomy. Overall, they found somewhat better relief of pain in the open group and a slightly greater rate of recurrence in the arthroscopic group. They identified subjects with early disease and with a preoperative arc of elbow flexion greater than 90° as a particularly favorable group for arthroscopic intervention.

TOTAL ELBOW ARTHROPLASTY

Total elbow replacement is an effective treatment for end-stage arthritis of the elbow. Total elbow

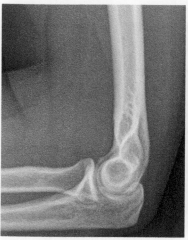
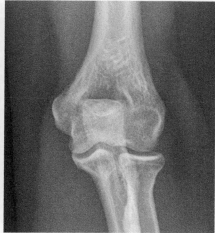

Fig. 1. A 41-year-old woman with new diagnosis of rheumatoid arthritis.

implants differ among several variables: degree of constraint (unconstrained, semiconstrained), cemented or uncemented, and short or long stems. Fully constrained (simple hinge) designs have been abandoned because of unacceptably high rates of loosening, as slight rotational and angular motions are transmitted as shear-stresses to the implant bone interface. In many series, with various surgical approaches, institutions, and types of prostheses, results have shown favorable relief of pain and improvement in elbow function.[10–19]

Elbow replacement surgery is not as reliable or durable as arthroplasty of the hip or knee. The elbow is the smallest large joint. The humerus and ulna are gracile and thin walled, and it has proven difficult to maintain stable fixation of a prosthesis in these bones compared with the hip, knee, and shoulder. In a recent review based on the Finnish arthroplasty registry, more than 1400

primary total elbow replacements were evaluated. They found the most common cause of failure was aseptic loosening. There was no difference in survival rates between different elbow designs. Stratifying between operations performed in specialty hospitals and in more unspecialized hospitals, they found about 1.5-fold increase in relative risk of failure.[20]

One might expect outcomes to be even worse in patients with rheumatoid arthritis, given the systemic implications of the disease and the fact that most patients are on immune-suppressing medications as part of ongoing medical treatment of their disease. In aggregate, it appears that total elbow replacements performed for rheumatoid arthritis are nearly as free of complications as those performed for other indications.[21] Some groups have reported good clinical results over fairly long follow-up using unlinked prostheses

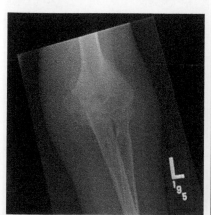
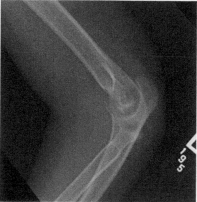

Fig. 2. Radiograph of a 47-year-old woman with longstanding systemic RA.

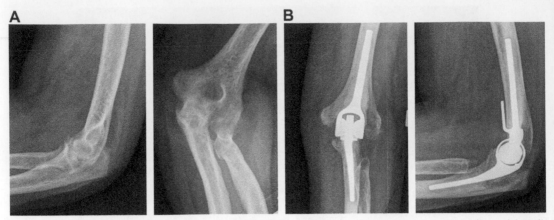

Fig. 3. (*A*) A 55-year-old man with longstanding systemic RA whose main affected joint was this elbow. (*B*) Radiograph at 3-year follow-up.

even in subjects with significant bone loss, some requiring bone graft augmentation at primary surgery.[22]

However, the decision to proceed to total elbow replacement should be taken lightly. It should be considered a last step because no other option is possible after elbow replacement other than a revision of the replacement. The question naturally arises when to choose that option. The conventional wisdom is not to do total elbow replacement in young patients. Celli and Morrey[23] reviewed 58 subjects who had undergone total elbow at less than 40 years of age and although they found a 22% revision rate by 91 months, the subjects were satisfied and had good functional outcomes at that point. There is also evidence that proceeding promptly to elbow replacement may improve outcome of this procedure. Results

of elbow replacement surgery in subjects who had a preceding rheumatoid surgery, either synovectomy or interposition arthroplasty, compared with those who did not has shown less favorable results. Interposition arthroplasty in particular was associated with greater risk of complication and failure in subsequent elbow replacement.[24]

MINI CASES
Case 1

A 41-year-old woman with new diagnosis of rheumatoid arthritis had elbow symptoms that were entirely synovitic; the synovitis caused what almost appeared to be a tense effusion (**Fig. 1**). The elbow motion was normal but painful at the extremes. She responded well to antiinflammatory medication.

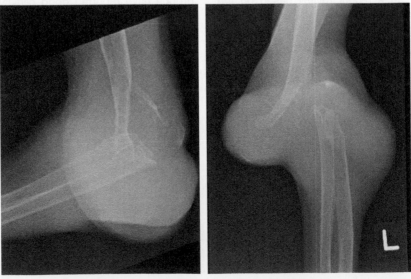

Fig. 4. Radiograph of a 70-year-old woman with severe, longstanding systemic RA.

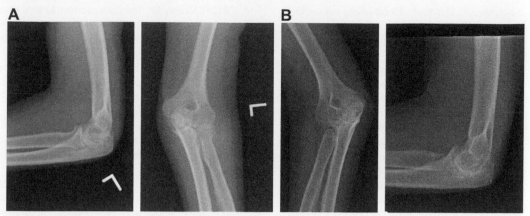

Fig. 5. (*A*) Radiograph of a 43-year-old right-hand dominant female office worker with RA. (*B*) Her follow-up radiograph at 7.5 years.

Case 2

A 47-year-old woman with longstanding systemic RA, including many prior surgeries in bilateral hands, knees, feet, and hips for RA, had elbows that have always hurt but recently had lost more stability and seemed unreliable to her (**Fig. 2**). Pain had been constant for years, and although it was severe she was used to it. The change she reacts to is the new worsening instability.

She declined to consider total elbow replacement because of unpleasant experiences with other joint arthroplasty. Focusing on her instability, she was treated with braces and occupational therapy and is doing well at medium-term follow-up.

Case 3

The main affected joint of this 55-year-old man with longstanding systemic RA was the elbow. The elbow was constantly painful and had lost motion (**Fig. 3**A). He was treated with a semicon-strained total elbow and is doing well at 3 years (see **Fig. 3**B).

Case 4

A 70-year-old woman with severe, longstanding systemic RA had many joints, including the elbow, that were mutilated by bone loss (**Fig. 4**). She understood that she would have been previously indicated for total elbow replacement, except that she refused because of negative experiences with right total elbow surgery that required revision and that still causes pain. She chose to continue local measures only, despite the complete insta-bility and quite severe pain of this condition.

Case 5

A 43-year-old right-hand dominant female office worker with RA (treated with methotrexate) who

had bilateral elbow pain, left worse than right, and who had bilateral total knee replacements was referred for total elbow replacement. On examina-tion she had more tenderness laterally and with forearm rotation than medial or with flexion exten-sion. The authors elected to pursue a synovectomy and radial head excision given her age, her radio-graphs (**Fig. 5**A), and the fact that she was still working. **Fig. 5**B is her follow-up radiograph at 7.5 years. Her pain relief was good over that time period except when she had systemic flares.

REFERENCES

1. Lehtinen JT, Kaarela K, Ikavalko M, et al. Incidence of elbow involvement in rheumatoid arthritis. A 15 year endpoint study. J Rheumatol 2001;28(1):70–4.
2. Abe A, Ishikawa H, Murasawa A, et al. Disease activity and the course of elbow joint deterioration over 10 years in the patients with early rheumatoid arthritis. Clin Rheumatol 2008;27(7):867–72.
3. Cunnington J, Marshall N, Hide G, et al. A randomized, double-blind, controlled study of ultrasound-guided corticosteroid injection into the joint of patients with inflammatory arthritis. Arthritis Rheum 2010;62(7):1862–9.
4. Bliddal H, Terslev L, Qvistgaard E, et al. A randomized, controlled study of a single intra-articular injection of etanercept or glucocorticoste-roids in patients with rheumatoid arthritis. Scand J Rheumatol 2006;35(5):341–5.
5. Fuerst M, Fink B, Ruther W. Survival analysis and long term results of elbow synovectomy in rheuma-toid arthritis. J Rheumatol 2006;33(5):892–6.
6. Nakagawa N, Abe S, Saegusa Y, et al. Long-term results of open elbow synovectomy for rheumatoid arthritis. Mod Rheumatol 2007;17(2):106–9.
7. Nemoto K, Arino H, Yoshihara Y, et al. Arthroscopic synovectomy for the rheumatoid elbow: a short-term

outcome. J Shoulder Elbow Surg 2004;13(6): 652–5.

8. Horiuchi K, Momohara S, Tomatsu T, et al. Arthroscopic synovectomy of the elbow in rheumatoid arthritis. J Bone Joint Surg Am 2002;84(3):342–7.

9. Tanaka N, Sakahashi H, Hirose K, et al. Arthroscopic and open synovectomy of the elbow in rheumatoid arthritis. J Bone Joint Surg Am 2006;88(3):521–5.

10. Cesar M, Roussanne Y, Bonnel F, et al. GSB III total elbow replacement in rheumatoid arthritis. J Bone Joint Surg Br 2007;89(3):330–4.

11. Amirfeyz R, Blewitt N. Mid-term outcome of GSB-III total elbow arthroplasty in patients with rheumatoid arthritis and patients with post-traumatic arthritis. Arch Orthop Trauma Surg 2009;129(11):1505–10.

12. Rauhaniemi J, Tiusanen H, Kyro A. Kudo total elbow arthroplasty in rheumatoid arthritis. Clinical and radiological results. J Hand Surg Br 2006;31(2):162–7.

13. Jensen CH, Jacobsen S, Ratchke M, et al. The GSB III elbow prosthesis in rheumatoid arthritis: a 2- to 9-year follow-up. Acta Orthop 2006;77(1):143–8.

14. van der Lugt JC, Geskus RB, Rozing PM. Primary Souter-Strathclyde total elbow prosthesis in rheumatoid arthritis. Surgical technique. J Bone Joint Surg Am 2005;87(Suppl 1(Pt 1)):67–77.

15. Khatri M, Stirrat AN. Souter-Strathclyde total elbow arthroplasty in rheumatoid arthritis: medium-term results. J Bone Joint Surg Br 2005;87(7):950–4.

16. Skytta ET, Remes V, Nietosvaara Y, et al. Similar results with 21 Kudo and 21 Souter-Strathclyde total elbow arthroplasties in patients with rheumatoid arthritis. Arch Orthop Trauma Surg 2008;128(10):1201–8.

17. Gill DR, Morrey BF. The Coonrad-Morrey total elbow arthroplasty in patients who have rheumatoid arthritis. A ten to fifteen-year follow-up study. J Bone Joint Surg Am 1998;80(9):1327–35.

18. Ewald FC, Simmons ED Jr, Sullivan JA, et al. Capitellocondylar total elbow replacement in rheumatoid arthritis. Long-term results. J Bone Joint Surg Am 1993;75(4):498–507.

19. Ovesen J, Olsen BS, Johannsen HV, et al. Capitellocondylar total elbow replacement in late-stage rheumatoid arthritis. J Shoulder Elbow Surg 2005;14(4): 414–20.

20. Skytta ET, Eskelinen A, Paavolainen P, et al. Total elbow arthroplasty in rheumatoid arthritis: a population-based study from the Finnish Arthroplasty Register. Acta Orthop 2009;80(4):472–7.

21. Cook C, Hawkins R, Aldridge JM 3rd, et al. Comparison of perioperative complications in patients with and without rheumatoid arthritis who receive total elbow replacement. J Shoulder Elbow Surg 2009; 18(1):21–6.

22. Mori T, Kudo H, Iwano K, et al. Kudo type-5 total elbow arthroplasty in mutilating rheumatoid arthritis: a 5- to 11-year follow-up. J Bone Joint Surg Br 2006; 88(7):920–4.

23. Celli A, Morrey BF. Total elbow arthroplasty in patients forty years of age or less. J Bone Joint Surg Am 2009;91(6):1414–8.

24. Fink B, Krey D, Schmielau G, et al. Results of elbow endoprostheses in patients with rheumatoid arthritis in correlation with previous operations. J Shoulder Elbow Surg 2002;11(4):360–7.

Current Concepts in the Treatment of Rheumatoid Arthritis of the Distal Radioulnar Joint

Peter M. Murray, MD

KEYWORDS

- Rheumatoid arthritis • Distal radioulnar joint
- Tendon rupture • Tenosynovectomy

Rheumatoid arthritis (RA) may progressively affect all articulations of the wrist. Involvement of the distal radioulnar joint (DRUJ) is common and may be the first clinical signs or symptoms of RA.[1,2] Patients may present to hand surgery with previously undiagnosed RA because of pain and disability of the DRUJ. When the DRUJ is affected by RA, upper extremity function can be notably affected, particularly when forearm rotation is compromised.

The anatomy and biomechanics of the DRUJ are complex, leading to predictable patterns of wrist deformity. Fixed instability of the DRUJ can develop in patients with RA, causing attritional rupture of the extensor tendons of the wrist. The potential for this profoundly compromising situation underscores the importance of regular evaluations by the hand surgeon or rheumatologist in order that upper extremity function in general, and wrist and digital function in particular, are closely monitored.

In patients with RA with extensive involvement, nonoperative measures are of nominal benefit. Operative intervention is generally indicated, particularly when advanced, nonremitting extensor tenosynovitis is present or when extensor tendon rupture has occurred. In these situations, tendon reconstruction must be coupled with salvage of the DRUJ by surgical means. In general, the DRUJ articulation is addressed in these patients by using one of 3 treatment principles: arthrodesis/pseudoarthrosis, resection, or arthroplasty. The development of the antitumor necrosis factor drugs have heralded a new and different generation of upper extremity RA deformity. These drugs have dramatically slowed the progression of this disease and potentially lessen DRUJ deformity for patients with RA.

ANATOMY AND BIOMECHANICS

In the forearm, the radius and ulna articulate through the proximal radioulnar joint (PRUJ) and DRUJ. The DRUJ consists of the sigmoid notch of the distal radius and the ulnar head that provides stability as a result of the bony (dorsal) and cartilaginous rims (volar) of the notch[3] Approximately 30% of DRUJ constraint is created by the articular contact between the ulnar head and sigmoid notch.

The sigmoid notch is shallow and concave and is located at the ulnar surface of radius epiphysis. The ulnar head is cylindrical with three-quarters of its surface covered in articular cartilage. The radius of curvature of the sigmoid notch is greater than the radius of curvature of the distal ulnar articular surface. The triangular fibrocartilage complex (TFCC) is the primary soft tissue stabilizer of the DRUJ. It is composed of the dorsal radioulnar ligament (DRUL) and volar radioulnar ligament (VRUL), the articular disc, the ulnotriquetral and ulnolunate ligaments, and the extensor carpi ulnaris (ECU) subsheath. The thickness of the TFCC articular disc is proportional to the degree of ulnar minus

Dr Murray has nothing to disclose and no funding support.
Department of Orthopedic Surgery, Mayo Clinic, 4500 San Pablo Road South, Jacksonville, FL 32224, USA
E-mail address: murray.peter@mayo.edu

Hand Clin 27 (2011) 49–55
doi:10.1016/j.hcl.2010.10.002

hand.theclinics.com

variance present on the posterior-anterior wrist radiograph.[4] The dorsal and volar DRUJ capsule is redundant, which permits translation of the radius relative to the ulna during normal forearm pronation and supination. The pronator quadratus is a dynamic stabilizer of the DRUJ.[5] It arises from the radial border of the distal radius and inserts along the ulnar border of the distal ulnar, just proximal to the DRUJ. It is composed of the deep and superficial heads and initiates pronation.

The forearm is a bicondylar joint articulating through both the proximal radioulnar joint and DRUJ. The axis of rotation passes from the radial head obliquely to the ulnar head and the normal range of motion is between 150 and 180°.[3,6] The difference in radius of curvature between the sigmoid notch and the ulnar head enables 4 to 6 mm of translation during pronation and supination[3,5,6] In pronation, the radius translates volar with respect to the ulnar, whereas in pronation it is reversed. This translation affects the congruency of the joint. Articular contact is greatest with zero degrees of forearm rotation and least at maximum supination or pronation.[3,6] By convention, instability of the DRUJ is described with the position of the ulna relative to the radius sigmoid notch. For instance, if the ulna is positioned dorsally, this is dorsal subluxation of the DRUJ even though the radius has migrated volar to the fixed ulna.

The DRUL and VRUL are the primarily soft tissue constraints responsible for stabilizing the DRUJ. These ligamentous constraints can become attenuated in patients with RA. Debate continues about which ligament provides the principal constraint to translation during pronation and supination.[3,6] Stuart and colleagues[7] contend that the VRUL tension peaks first during pronation, preventing dorsal translation of the ulna, whereas the DRUL tension peaks in a similar fashion and prevents volar translation of the ulnar in supination. Dynamic stability of the DRUJ is provided by both the pronator quadratus and the ECU tendon[5,8] The 2 heads of the pronator quadratus provide convergence stability of the DRUJ and contraction of the ECU tendon depresses the ulna volarly. The interosseous membrane also provides convergence stability.

DIAGNOSIS AND IMAGING

First described by Vaughn-Jackson in 1948, the classic presentation of DRUJ disruption along with rupture of the extensor digiti minimi quinti (EDQM) and extensor digitorum comminus (EDC) to ring and small finger resulting in small finger and ring finger metacarpophalangeal (MCP) extension lag, is known as the Vaughn-Jackson syndrome and may be the first indication of previously undiagnosed RA (**Figs. 1** and **2**).[9] Patients with RA may first manifest the condition with a painful DRUJ with overlying synovitis. The finding that may bring the patient to the hand surgeon, whether directly or following an evaluation by a primary care physician, is extensor tenosynovitis nonresponsive to medical management. It is important for the hand surgeon to carefully examine the DRUJ for instability, as well as to assess the range of motion of the forearm. Any pain with forearm rotation should be noted. Instability may be identified as a clunk of the ulnar head subluxing or dislocating from the sigmoid notch of the radius then relocating back. Limitations in range of forearm rotation or persistent instability of the DRUJ can notably alter patient's abilities to perform activities of daily living. These patients may present with a prominent, dorsally subluxed or dislocated and fixed ulna relative to the radius. Alternatively, the patient may present with a rupture of the EDQM or the EDC to small and ring fingers. Patients with a ruptured EDQM are unable to demonstrate independent extension of the small finger, but may have the ability to extend the small finger through use of the EDC in concert with activation of the other digital extensors. In most circumstances, the EDQM and the EDC to the small finger are both ruptured and the patient has an extension lag to the small finger at the MCP joint.

Sequentially, each digit is evaluated for integrity of its EDC tendon and for the presence of extension lag. Extension lag may be the first indication of EDC dysfunction. The range of motion of the MCP joint should be compared with the contralateral side because MCP articular disorders can also limit MCP motion. The overlying soft tissues should be evaluated because some rheumatoid patients may develop markedly thin dystrophic skin following

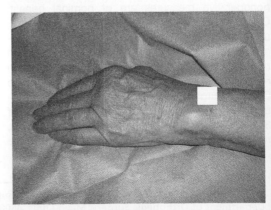

Fig. 1. Clinical presentation of the caput ulna syndrome with the dorsal prominence of the distal ulna.

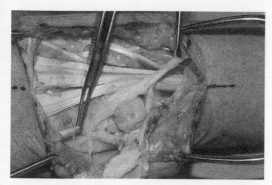

Fig. 2. Intraoperative demonstration of the caput ulna syndrome with prominent dorsal positioning of the distal ulnar head. Also seen is rupture of the EDQM and EDC to ring tendons.

prolonged treatment with oral corticosteroids. It is imperative for the examiner to assess the function of the ipsilateral elbow and shoulder as well as the function of the ipsilateral median, radial, and ulnar nerves. RA affecting the elbow or shoulder may alter upper extremity usage and preempt hand and wrist surgery. A detailed neurologic examination of the motor and sensory function of the ulnar and median nerves, as well as the motor function of the radial nerve, should be assessed and documented. Sensory testing with Semmes Weinstein monofilaments is a reliable threshold testing tool. Typically, soft tissue instability of the DRUJ is not a clinical issue for patients with RA because bone and joint destruction outpaces soft tissue problems. In addition, isolated triangular fibrocartilage complex abnormality is generally not a clinical problem for these patients. The patient's cervical spine should be evaluated for atlantoaxial instability and subaxial instability. This assessment should include reflex testing along with the motor and sensory testing

described earlier. The combination of limited neck flexion, extension or rotation with pain, or upper extremity parasthesias should alert the examiner to the potential of cervical spine instability and the need for further evaluation.

Imaging of the DRUJ in the patient with RA is generally limited to posteroanterior (PA) and lateral radiographs of the wrist. In patients with advanced RA involving the DRUJ, concentric narrowing of the DRUJ articulation is seen with erosion of the sigmoid notch, the ulnar head, or both. These radiographic features are generally seen in the context of the typical radiocarpal joint changes of RA (**Fig. 3**). For persisting extensor tenosynovitis refractory to medical management, magnetic resonance imaging (MRI) may be helpful in assessing the extent of the extensor tendon involvement, but this is generally not necessary in lieu of a thorough physical examination of the wrist. Likewise, extensor tendon dysfunction or rupture is typically diagnosed on physical examination and MRI is seldom required.

TREATMENT AND OUTCOME
Nonoperative Management

Nonoperative treatment of RA of the DRUJ may provide brief intervals of symptomatic relief. Initially, splintage and activity restriction may prove helpful, particularly if the patient is experiencing an acute flare of RA. A long arm splint with the elbow at 90°, the forearm neutral, and wrist and hand in the resting, prehensile position is preferred. The splint may be worn at any time the patient experiences symptoms, but is generally recommended at bedtime. Avoidance of activities that irritate the DRUJ, such as forceful supination or pronation, will likely help to control the patient's symptoms. Injections of a small quantity of corticosteroid

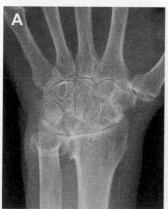
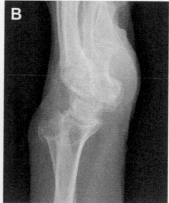

Fig. 3. PA (*A*) and lateral radiograph (*B*) of patient with RA of the wrist. Note the concentric cartilage shadow narrowing of the radiocarpal, midcarpal, and DRUJs. There is notable ulnar translation of the carpus.

medication mixed with a local anesthetic may be effective for longer-term relief when placed in the DRUJ proper using fluoroscopic guidance. Injections into overlying proliferative tenosynovium is advised when the tenosynovium has been recalcitrant to appropriate medical management and before the consideration of surgical extensor tenosynovectomy. In most circumstances, patients have already been treated with antiinflammatory medications or various RA remitting agents such as etanercept (Enbrel) or infliximab (Remicade) such that additional medications would likely prove ineffective. Patients should be evaluated and followed by a rheumatologist, particularly in the setting of a previously undiagnosed RA.

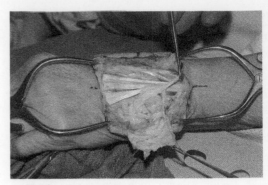

Fig. 4. Elevation of the extensor retinaculum exposing the contents of the third, fourth, and fifth dorsal compartments.

Tenosynovectomy

When extensor tenosynovitis is not resolved by appropriate medical therapy along with other nonoperative measures, surgical extensor tenosynovectomy with or without DRUJ reconstruction should be considered. In most circumstances, and assuming that the patient is otherwise medically fit for surgery, persisting tenosynovectomy should be addressed surgically if not resolved following 3 to 4 months of appropriate medical therapy. This surgery is undertaken to prevent future extensor tendon rupture. In some situations, rupture of EDQM or EDC to small or ring fingers may have already occurred (see **Fig. 2**).

For wrist extensor tenosynovectomy, a dorsal longitudinal midline incision over the radiocarpal joint is preferred. The soft tissues are carefully elevated as radial and ulnar full-thickness flaps, being careful to protect the integrity of the skin, which is often dystrophic in these patients. The radial and ulnar sensory nerves are carefully protected as well. Although the extensor tenosynovitis may only be involving the fifth and sixth dorsal compartments of the wrist, in most circumstances, tenosynovitis may also be found in the fourth or even the third dorsal compartment. Therefore, a complete dorsal wrist extensor tenosynovectomy is generally preformed. The extensor retinaculum is elevated in a radial to ulnar fashion off the Lister tubercle (**Fig. 4**). Sequentially, the extensor pollicis longus, the extensor indicis proprius, the EDC to index, long, ring, and small fingers, and the EDQM are delivered, examined for rupture, and a tenosynovectomy performed. The sixth dorsal compartment containing the ECU tendon is inspected and tenosynovium removed only as necessary. If the sixth dorsal compartment is surgically violated, it is important to preserve, if possible, the ECU subsheath. Failure to do so could result in ECU instability.

If extensor tendon ruptures are present, reconstruction is performed by a side-to-side tendon transfer in most instances. For example, a ruptured EDQM can be reconstructed by a side-to-side tendon transfer to the adjacent EDC to ring and an EDQM and an EDC to ring tendon transfer can be reconstructed by a side-to-side tendon transfer to the EDC to long. If the EDC to long is also ruptured, it is advisable to transfer the EDC to long to the EDC to index while transferring the extensor indicis proprius tendon to the EDC to ring and the EDQM using a Pulvertaft technique.[3]

When extensor tendon ruptures have occurred, the attrition of the tendon over time prohibits end-to-end tendon repair. Furthermore, it is necessary to remove whatever bony excrescence that is the cause for tendon abrasive wear to prevent further tendon ruptures. At time of surgery, surgeon and patient should be prepared to proceed with one of several reconstructive options for the DRUJ. These options can be divided into 2 categories of surgery: resection surgery or arthrodesis/pseudoarthrosis surgery.

Postoperative rehabilitation following tendon transfer surgery requires immobilization of the affected MCP joint and the radiocarpal joint in extension for 4 weeks. An attractive alternative to this in the patient with RA is the use of an extension outrigger splint immobilizing the wrist and affected MCP joints in extension while allowing progressive active flexion with passive extension. After complete immobilization the first postoperative week, this construct permits 0 to 30° in the second postoperative weeks, 0 to 60° in the third postoperative week, then full active flexion in the fourth postoperative week before discontinuing the splint. Immobilization and rehabilitation of the radiocarpal joint and the DRUJ may be further modified depending on whether bony procedures were performed concurrently.

Darrach Procedure

Although Severinus first reported resection of the distal ulna, the procedure has become known as the Darrach procedure.[1] In 1912, Darrach[10] described his experience with the procedure for treatment of patients with so-called anterior dislocation of the ulna. The Darrach procedure is indicated in patients who are low demand and elderly, such as patients with caput ulna syndrome from RA. Poor results have been reported in the young, more active patient.[11]

The Darrach procedure is a resection of the distal ulna with the level of resection located 1 to 2 cm proximal to the most proximal extent of the sigmoid notch of the distal radius (**Figs. 5** and **6**). This level of resection may help avoid convergence of the distal radius and ulna because this level of resection is just proximal to the pronator quadratus. It is useful to preserve the TFCC during resection of the distal ulna. Several stabilization procedures have been described for the distal ulna stump. Breen and Jupiter[12] described a combined tenodesis of the distal ulnar stump using both the ECU and flexor carpi ulnaris, weaved through the distal ulnar.

In general, the Darrach procedure is an effective procedure in the patient with RA of the wrist. Rana and Taylor[13] reported 93% pain relief and 87% restoration of forearm rotation in their patients with RA. Fraser and colleagues[14] underscored the superiority of results with the Darrach procedure in the rheumatoid patient compared with the nonrheumatoid patient. They found that 86% of the patients with RA were satisfied following the distal ulna resection compared with only 36% of the patients with osteoarthritis. Thirupathi and colleagues[15] showed in a series of 38 patients with RA at 7.4 years follow-up from distal ulna resection that ulnar translocation of the carpus occurred in 44% of patients. This and other studies have led to the opinion that removal of the ulna can lead to progressive ulnar translation of the carpus.

Sauvé-Kapandji Procedure

The Sauvé-Kapandji procedure involves arthrodesis of the DRUJ while enabling forearm rotation by the creation of a pseudarthrosis just proximal to the DRUJ.[16] Theoretically, this procedure has the advantage of maintenance of bony support of the ulnar carpus through retention of the distal ulna. Whether the Sauvé-Kapandji procedure arrests ulnar translation of the carpus is controversial.[1,17] The procedure is performed by debridement of eburnated bone from the articular surfaces of the DRUJ to create matched cancellous surfaces for arthrodesis with either parallel K-wires or a cannulated cancellous screw for stabilization. The ulnar head is positioned in 1 to 2 mm of negative variance to avoid ulnar impaction. If K-wires are chosen, the 0.0625-mm variety is preferred. The surgeon should use 2 K-wires placed parallel to each other and perpendicular to the axis of the ulna head and radius. Also, the K-wires should breach the far cortices of the radial styloid process to allow retrieval should the K-wire break. However, the K-wire advancement through the opposite cortex should not be to such an extent that the overlying soft tissues are jeopardized. Alternatively, a 3.5-mm cannulated cortical or cancellous screw can be used depending on the adequacy of the bone, and applied in a fashion that provides compression of the debrided DRUJ surfaces. The compression of the surfaces can be achieved by countersinking the screw head using an overdrilling technique of the near cortical surface. At the same time, a 1-cm resection of the ulnar shaft just proximal to the level of the sigmoid notch enables forearm rotation. Symptomatic instability of the proximal ulna stump can possibly result and require stabilization of the stump performed by tenodesis using the ECU/FCU technique previously mentioned for the Darrach resection.[12] The need for using autologous bone graft or an allograft material in the DRUJ arthrodesis is debated.

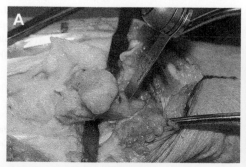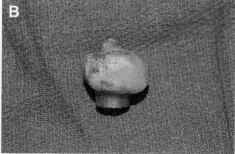

Fig. 5. Exposed distal ulna showed the location of planned resection (*A*). Resected distal ulna from a patient undergoing a Darrach procedure (*B*).

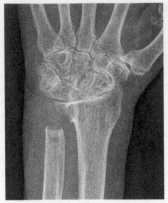

Fig. 6. Radiographic appearance of the wrist following a Darrach procedure.

Outcomes of the Sauvé-Kapandji procedure have been documented by Goncalves[18] as consistently better than those of the Darrach in 22 patients. Taleisnik[19] described elimination of pain, restoration of forearm rotation, and few complications in 37 patients with the Sauvé-Kapandji procedure. Many question whether the Sauvé-Kapandji prevents the progression of ulnar translocation of the wrist.[1,17]

Hemiresection Interposition Arthroplasty Procedure

The hemiresection interposition technique (HIT) arthroplasty was originally reported by Bowers[20] for patients with RA. In this procedure, the radial portion of the distal ulnar head is resected while preserving the foveal attachments of the TFCC and ulnar styloid. Capsular flaps as well as the pronator quadratus are used for interposition between the radius and the ulna. This procedure can be effective for restoring function and relieving pain in patients with RA affecting the DRUJ.

The matched distal ulnar resection described by Watson and Gabuzda[21] is a similar technique of resection of the radial portion of the ulnar head and may be considered a modification of the original Bowers technique. However, in this technique, the ulna is contoured to match the morphology of the ulnar aspect of the radius to lessen the possibility of convergence instability of the ulna on the radius.

Bowers[20] reported good results with the hemiresection interposition arthroplasty in 27 patients with mild RA and minimal destructive joint changes. Watson and Gabuzda[21] reported good results in 34 patients with matched distal ulnar resection and RA. Despite the reported success of these procedures in patients with RA using the Bowers hemiresection interposition arthroplasty as well as the matched distal ulnar resection described by

Watson and Gabuzda,[21] neither are currently considered first-line surgical solutions for patients with painful, disrupted DRUJs from RA.[1]

FUTURE DIRECTIONS

Arthroplasty of the DRUJ is a potential new option for reconstruction of the DRUJ, thanks to considerable product development activity in the past 10 years. Larger, better controlled clinical studies with longer follow-up are needed to further evaluate these devices. In general, DRUJ arthroplasty is reserved for failures following distal ulnar resection and is not currently considered a primary reconstruction tool for patients with RA of the DRUJ. The use of a metallic prosthetic distal ulna endoprostheses can restore the mechanical integrity of the forearm as well as the stability of the DRUJ. DRUJ implant arthroplasty with sigmoid notch implants have also been developed, although long-term follow-up has not been reported.[6] A series of 19 DRUJ arthroplasties (17 patients) using an ulnar head endoprosthesis has been reported with 2-year follow-up[22] Overall pain scores decreased by 50%, grip strength improved by 16%, forearm rotation was unchanged, and all wrists were stable. Scheker and colleagues[23] published their results using a ball and socket DRUJ total joint arthroplasty that allows translation between the native radius and the ulna component. They reported on 23 patients with follow-up at a mean of 15 months. Complete pain relief and normal forearm rotation was reported in all patients. In a later report by the investigators, 31 patients had follow-up at 5.9 years with similar results.[24]

The future will likely lead clinicians away from surgical reconstruction of the wrist as RA is diagnosed earlier and medical management becomes more and more effective at controlling the disease. Genomics may enable the identification of susceptible individuals for RA, whether the ultimate diagnosis is seronegative or seropositive disease. With early detection followed by treatment with anti–tumor necrosis factor drugs, it is likely that rheumatoid wrist surgery in general, and rheumatoid DRUJ reconstruction in particular, will become unusual, if not preventable, except in populations that are underserved or have no access to medical care.

REFERENCES

1. Lee SK, Hausman MR. Management of the distal radioulnar joint in rheumatoid arthritis. Hand Clin 2005; 21(4):577–89.

2. Leak RS, Rayan GM, Arthur RE. Longitudinal radiographic analysis of rheumatoid arthritis in

the hand and wrist. J Hand Surg Am 2003;28(3): 427–34.

3. Adams B. Distal radioulnar joint instability. In: Green D, Hotchkiss R, Pederson W, et al, editors. Operative hand surgery. 5th edition. Churchill Livingstone; 2005. p. 605–44.

4. Werner FW, Palmer AK, Fortino MD, et al. Force transmission through the distal ulna: effect of ulnar variance, lunate fossa angulation, and radial and palmar tilt of the distal radius. J Hand Surg Am 1992;17(3):423–8.

5. Szabo RM. Distal radioulnar joint instability. Instr Course Lect 2007;56:79–89.

6. Murray P, Adams J, Lam J, et al. Disorders of the distal radioulnar joint. Instr Course Lect 2010;59: 295–311.

7. Stuart PR, Berger RA, Linscheid RL, et al. The dorsopalmar stability of the distal radioulnar joint. J Hand Surg Am 2000;25(4):689–99.

8. Stuart PR. Pronator quadratus revisited. J Hand Surg Br 1996;21(6):714–22.

9. Vaughan-Jackson O. Rheumatoid hand deformities considered in the light of tendon imbalance. J Bone Joint Surg Br 1962;44-B(4):764–75.

10. Darrach W. Anterior dislocation of the head of the ulna. Ann Surg 1912;56:802–3.

11. Bieber EJ, Linscheid RL, Dobyns JH, et al. Failed distal ulna resections. J Hand Surg Am 1988;13(2): 193–200.

12. Breen TF, Jupiter JB. Extensor carpi ulnaris and flexor carpi ulnaris tenodesis of the unstable distal ulna. J Hand Surg Am 1989;14(4):612–7.

13. Rana NA, Taylor AR. Excision of the distal end of the ulna in rheumatoid arthritis. J Bone Joint Surg Br 1973;55(1):96–105.

14. Fraser KE, Diao E, Peimer CA, et al. Comparative results of resection of the distal ulna in rheumatoid arthritis and post-traumatic conditions. J Hand Surg Br 1999;24(6):667–70.

15. Thirupathi RG, Ferlic DC, Clayton ML. Dorsal wrist synovectomy in rheumatoid arthritis–a long-term study. J Hand Surg Am 1983;8(6):848–56.

16. Sauve L, Kapandji M. Nouvelle technique de traitement chirurgical des luxations récidivantes isolées de l'extrémité inferieure du cubitus. J Chir 1936;47: 589–94.

17. Feldon P, Terrono A, Nalebuff E, et al. Rheumatoid arthritis and other connective tissue diseases. In: Green D, Hotchkiss R, Pederson C, et al, editors. Green's operative hand surgery, vol. 2. Philadelphia: Churchill Livingstone; 2005. p. 2049–136.

18. Goncalves D. Correction of disorders of the distal radio-ulnar joint by artificial pseudarthrosis of the ulna. J Bone Joint Surg Br 1974;56B(3):462–4.

19. Taleisnik J. The Sauve-Kapandji procedure. Clin Orthop Relat Res 1992;275:110–23.

20. Bowers WH. Distal radioulnar joint arthroplasty: the hemiresection-interposition technique. J Hand Surg Am 1985;10(2):169–78.

21. Watson HK, Gabuzda GM. Matched distal ulna resection for posttraumatic disorders of the distal radioulnar joint. J Hand Surg Am 1992;17(4): 724–30.

22. Willis AA, Berger RA, Cooney WP 3rd. Arthroplasty of the distal radioulnar joint using a new ulnar head endoprosthesis: preliminary report. J Hand Surg Am 2007;32(2):177–89.

23. Scheker LR, Babb BA, Killion PE. Distal ulnar prosthetic replacement. Orthop Clin North Am 2001; 32(2):365–76, x.

24. Laurentin-Perez LA, Goodwin AN, Babb BA, et al. A study of functional outcomes following implantation of a total distal radioulnar joint prosthesis. J Hand Surg Eur Vol 2008;33(1):18–28.

Current Concepts and Treatment for the Rheumatoid Wrist

Marco Rizzo, MD[a],*, William P. Cooney III, MD[a,b]

KEYWORDS

- Rheumatoid arthritis • Arthrodesis • Arthroplasty • Wrist

Rheumatoid arthritis (RA) is an autoimmune-mediated process that results in joint destruction, deformity, and pain. Due to the systemic nature of the disease, it routinely affects multiple joints. The severity of the condition may be widely variable. In severe cases, RA can lead to a significant amount of joint destruction and deformity as compared with osteoarthritis.

The inflammatory process targets the synovium, tenosynovium, and cartilage, resulting in damage to the joints, adjacent soft tissues, and bone. The etiology remains somewhat unclear, but it appears to be linked to a neutrophil infiltration, which leads to the release of free radicals and lysosomal enzymes and results in damage to local tissues. The activation appears to be mediated (at least in part) by activation of the HLA-II locus.[1]

Wrist involvement in RA is common. Within 2 years of diagnosis, more than half of patients will have wrist pain, and more than 90% will have wrist disease by 10 years.[2] Although wrist involvement is generally thought to be less disabling than RA of the fingers and hand, it can be a significant cause of pain and disability. Severe disease with bony destruction and synovitis in the wrist can also result in soft-tissue problems including tendon ruptures.[3,4]

In addition to musculoskeletal involvement, systemic manifestations of RA can occur. Felty syndrome can result in a low white blood count and splenomegaly in association with RA. Still syndrome can involve children or adults and results in fevers, rash, and arthritis. The heart, blood vessels, lungs, and skin may also be affected in patients with RA.

DIAGNOSIS AND EVALUATION

Synovitis is the major clinical feature of RA (**Fig. 1**). Pain and functional limitation are typically the primary reasons patients present for evaluation. Occasionally patients present to the physician because they are concerned about deformity and clinical appearance. A complete medical history including that of RA is essential. The evaluation should include history of previous surgery and all medications. Past experiences with surgery for RA will shed significant light on future possible pitfalls and/or successes. A complete examination from the neck to the hand is extremely important, remembering that cervical spine disease is not uncommon in RA. A complete workup includes radiographs of the cervical spine and electromyography in patients with radicular or neurologic symptoms. Systemic evaluation of the musculoskeletal system will round off an appropriate workup of these often complex patients. Establishing a relationship with the patient's rheumatologist is important to better understand the patient, his or her disease, and operative planning when necessary. In addition, if the patient has lower extremity disease, it is advisable to address this issue before major upper extremity reconstruction or surgery because the patient will likely require crutch assistance for their lower extremity recovery.

Pain and synovitis of the elbow can affect the proximal and distal radioulnar joints and the forearm axis of rotation. In addition, synovitis of the elbow can result in posterior interosseous nerve dysfunction that can mimic tendon ruptures of

a Department of Orthopedic Surgery, Mayo Clinic, 200 First Street SW, Rochester, MN 55905, USA
b Pro-sports, Hand and Upper Extremity, 1355 37th Street, Suite 301, Vero Beach, FL 32960, USA
* Corresponding author.
E-mail address: rizzo.marco@mayo.edu

Hand Clin 27 (2011) 57–72
doi:10.1016/j.hcl.2010.09.004
0749-0712/11/$ — see front matter © 2011 Elsevier Inc. All rights reserved.

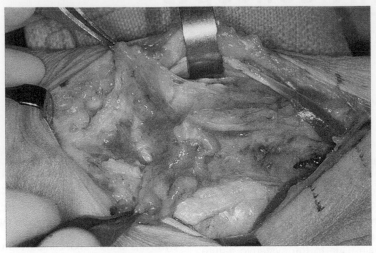

Fig. 1. Note the extensive synovitis in this patient. An extended longitudinal approach to the wrist allows for complete dorsal tenosynovectomy and synovectomy.

the hand. Synovitis of the wrist will affect the appearance of the hand and its function. Dorsal synovitis is generally more readily noted than volar synovitis because of the more superficial position of the dorsal synovium. The prestyloid recess of the ulna is a hypervascular area and is commonly affected in RA. This involvement can result in cartilage destruction and attenuation of the stabilizing ligaments, leading to dorsal displacement of the ulna and the caput ulna syndrome.[5] Although less obvious, volar wrist synovitis and inflammation may be extensive. Unfortunately, the initial presenting sign may be attritional flexor tendon rupture secondary to the synovitis, bony destruction, and osteophytosis of the carpus.[3] In long-standing or severe disease, the supporting soft tissues of the wrist become progressively incompetent and the wrist deforms. As a result, the carpus translates ulnarly and supinates, resulting in radial deviation of the wrist; this significantly contributes to the classic zig-zag deformity of the wrist-hand complex (see **Fig. 1**).[6]

Clinical evaluation of the wrist includes assessment of pain, degree of swelling, range of motion, grip and pinch strength, deformity, stability, and crepitus. Tenderness is usually most notable at areas of maximal swelling and joint destruction. Pain with resisted flexion and extension will reflect not only joint disease, but may also suggest tenosynovitis and potential "tendons at risk." Assessing passive versus active motion is helpful and may reflect the source of pathology—failure to actively extend a digit may be secondary to tendon rupture.[7] However, other causes may be the culprit, for example, volar subluxation of the metacarpophalangeal (MP) joint, extensor tendon

subluxation due to sagittal band insufficiency, or posterior interosseous neuropathy at the elbow. Common RA presentations include compression neuropathy of the wrist, as is seen in carpal tunnel syndrome, resulting from direct inflammatory influence on the nerve as well as tenosynovitis, synovitis, and joint destruction of the carpus. Carpal tunnel release usually combines with flexor tenosynovectomy in patients with RA, and generally carries a favorable prognosis.[8] Patients with bilateral and multiple upper extremity joint involvement pose special challenges, and prioritization of the patient's complaints and dysfunction. The skin in patients with RA is typically thin at high risk of ulceration. Problems can occur with wound healing. Rheumatoid nodules may be present and can often be painful, and are associated with joint deformity.

Radiographs of the wrist are important in discerning the degree of bony destruction and arthritis. Radiographs are critical for operative planning and to help determine what can and cannot be done from a surgical standpoint. Joint space narrowing is most commonly noted as the early finding at the distal radioulnar and the radioscaphoid joints.[9,10] Mid-carpal radiographic disease is typically a later finding.[11,12] Radiographic findings are also the basis for some of the more commonly used classification systems.[13,14] The classification of Larsen and colleagues[14] is not specific to the wrist but is commonly used (**Table 1**). This classification is based on stages 0 to 5, with stage 0 being a normal joint and stage 5 revealing a mutilated or ankylosed joint. The Wrightington classification is specific to the wrist and ranges from stages 1 to 4.[13]

Table 1
The Larsen classification of rheumatoid arthritis based on radiographs

Larsen Stage	Radiographic Appearance
0	Normal joint
1	Periarticular swelling, osteoporosis, slight narrowing
2	Erosion and mild joint space narrowing
3	Moderate destructive changes and joint space narrowing
4	End-stage destruction, preservation of articular surface
5	Mutilating disease, destruction of normal articular surfaces

From Larsen A, Dale K, Eek M. Radiographic evaluation of rheumatoid arthritis and related conditions by standard reference films. Acta Radiol Diagn (Stockh) 1977;18: 481–91; with permission.

In addition to radiographic assessment, the system outlines treatment recommendations based on the stage of disease. Stage 1 radiographs demonstrate osteoporosis, with cysts and erosions, and the recommended treatment is synovectomy. In stage 2 disease, radiographs reveal carpal instability; the recommended treatment is soft-tissue stabilization or partial arthrodesis of the wrist. By stage 3, the wrist has frank destruction and subluxation, and these patients likely require an arthroplasty or arthrodesis. In stage 4 disease, radiographs show severe radius destruction, and these wrists are generally restricted to arthrodesis as the only practical treatment option. Simmen and Huber[15] proposed an alternate classification system, not based so much on radiographs but rather more on the natural course of the disease. Type 1 is defined as the ankylosing type, characterized by spontaneous fusion of the wrist. Type 2 is the osteoarthritic type, and has characteristics of osteoarthritis and osteoporosis. These patients tend to have some inherent wrist stability. Type 3 patients are defined as the disintegrative type, and have significant bone loss and instability; they are subdivided into type 3a (more ligamentous instability) and type 3b (more bony resorption).

Additional radiographs may be helpful. Computed tomography provides a more precise sense of the degree of arthritic and joint involvement. Magnetic resonance imaging (MRI) better clarifies the degree of soft-tissue synovitis and tenosynovitis as well as the bony architecture. MR images have revealed improvement in tenosynovitis in response to treatment.[16] Scoring systems based on MRI have been proposed to grade the cartilage changes in patients with early RA.[17] In addition, in patients with early RA, bone edema on MRI has been shown to predict patients who go on to develop radiographic damage, and may help identify patients who could benefit from more aggressive treatment.[18]

NONOPERATIVE TREATMENT

Static and dynamic splinting is an established treatment for pain relief, functional improvement, and hopeful correction of deformity. In 2003, A Cochrane Database review showed that although patients seem to prefer wearing splints to not wearing them, there is no proven benefit with respect to pain or range of motion.[19] Veehof and colleagues[20] showed that wearing wrist splints for as little as 4 weeks can significantly help with pain. However, function and patient-related outcome measures were not significantly different when compared with controls. Another prospective randomized study showed that static resting splinting in the treatment of early RA does not significantly improve function and pain or retard deformity progression when compared with placebo.[21]

Intra-articular injection of steroid has been shown to improve swelling, pain, and patient-perceived outcomes.[22] In a prospective randomized trial, Konai and colleagues[23] concluded that intra-articular steroid injection was superior to systemic corticosteroid in treatment of monoarticular RA of the knee. More specific to the wrist, Weitoft and Ronnblom[24] prospectively evaluated the use of splinting as an adjunct following steroid injection of the wrist, and found no difference in outcomes between the groups. These investigators went on to caution against assuming other joints affected by RA will respond in a similar fashion to knees. More recent investigations have included the use of intra-articular injection of anti–tumor necrosis factor (TNF) agents, and have determined that it is generally safe.[25] Bliddal and colleagues[26] compared the use of intra-articular wrist injections of 25 mg enteracept versus 40 mg of methylprednisolone in a randomized trial. Results revealed no significant difference in outcomes. The investigators concluded that due to the cost of enteracept, it should be reserved primarily for patients who have adverse effects to steroid injections.

Multiple pharmacologic treatments have been used to subdue the inflammatory process of RA. Medications such as corticosteroids and methotrexate have been prescribed for years. Many surgeons prefer stopping noncorticosteroid anti-inflammatory medications for a period before and following surgery to help avoid delayed healing and infection.[27] Other studies have shown that continuing methotrexate does not increase the risk of perioperative infection.[28] Newer generation medications including anti-TNF agents have shown promise in ameliorating the synovitis and disease progression of RA. This advance has fortuitously led to fewer patients requiring surgical intervention and improved outcomes after such treatment. However, the medications have been shown to increase generalized infection rates especially in the lower respiratory tract and soft tissues, and particularly in patients who are also on corticosteroids,[29] and perioperative risk, especially for orthopedic procedures, is still forthcoming. Previous studies suggest no increase risk of the use of infliximab in patients undergoing surgery for Crohn disease.[30] The impact of the medications on perioperative morbidity, if any, has yet to be fully realized. These agents vary in the time taken to be cleared from the bloodstream, for example, 8 days for enteracept, 15 days for adalimumab, and 57 days for infliximab. At present, most surgeons in consultation with patients and their rheumatologists are stopping these medications perioperatively.

OPERATIVE TREATMENT

Considerations for surgery of the rheumatoid wrist require a thoughtful assessment of many factors. These patients require a comprehensive evaluation. Persons affected by RA may be nutritionally depleted as a result of their disease as well as the medications used for treatment. Thus, nutritional assessment and optimization is important. It is also important to appreciate that the poor pharmacologic control of the disease can undermine the outcome following surgery. Anesthetic risk is higher in patients with cervical spine disease.

The timing and indication for surgery remain somewhat controversial.[31] Persistent symptoms, synovitis, or swelling despite a 3- to 6-month course of conservative treatment can be viewed by most physicians as an indication for surgery.[32,33] Exceptions include cases in which surgery would be prophylactic against irreversible soft-tissue injury or damage such as is seen in tendon ruptures. Deformity, or progression of deformity of the wrist, such as a zig-zag deformity, has been advocated by some surgeons as requiring prophylactic intervention.[34,35] Frank tendon rupture itself is generally an indication for surgery.

Contraindications for surgery include significant comorbidities and poor general health. Poor or insufficient proximal arm function that is not correctable is a relative contraindication to wrist surgery. Relative contraindications for wrist arthroplasty (including total wrist replacement) include history of previous infection, insufficient bone stock, and long-standing fixed wrist deformity.

Surgical treatments for the rheumatoid wrist generally include synovectomy, tenosynovectomy, tendon repair/reconstruction, treatment of the arthritic distal radioulnar joint, partial and complete arthrodesis of the radiocarpal joint, and wrist arthroplasty. Multiple procedures are commonly done in the same setting.

SYNOVECTOMY AND TENOSYNOVECTOMY
Dorsal Synovectomy and Tenosynovectomy

Indications for synovectomy include patients with fairly well preserved wrist motion, moderate swelling and relative absence of joint disease. Dorsal wrist synovectomy and tenosynovectomy have been shown to improve pain and swelling in patients with RA.[36–38] Synovectomy of the wrist can be performed through a dorsal approach to the wrist (**Fig. 2**). The retinaculum is elevated from the fourth or fourth-fifth compartment interval, and appropriate flaps are raised to reveal the extensor tendons. Tenosynovectomy may then be performed, and the wrist capsule is visualized deep to the tendons. A posterior interosseous neurectomy can be performed deep to the fourth compartment tendons at the level of the distal radius just proximal to the radiocarpal joint. The distal radioulnar joint (DRUJ) is exposed deep to the fifth compartment, and the radiocarpal joint can be exposed through a ligament-sparing approach to facilitate synovectomy. Stabilization of the DRUJ is often recommended after synovectomy. Bone disease and spurs when present can also be removed from the carpus, distal ulna, and radius. Although most surgeons prefer an open approach for dorsal synovectomy, an arthroscopic technique has also been proposed.[39,40] Advantages of the arthroscopic technique include less morbidity, limited dissection, and improved postoperative motion. However, indications for the arthroscopic approach are limited to patients with isolated wrist disease and absence of tenosynovial involvement. Studies have shown that although short-term benefits of early synovectomy are fairly reliable, it does not necessarily correlate with long-term disease progression and retardation of joint destruction.[41,42]

Additional procedures can be performed in conjunction with dorsal synovectomy. In patients

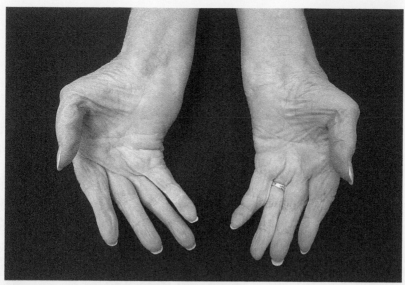

Fig. 2. A 68-year-old woman with long-standing rheumatoid arthritis. The wrist has collapsed into radial deviation, which has contributed to ulnar drift of the fingers resulting in the classic zig-zag deformity of the wrist-hand complex.

with significant wrist collapse, lengthening or transfer of the extensor carpi radialis longus (ERCL) tendon to the extensor carpi ulnaris (ECU) tendon can help correct the radial deviation of the wrist and the ulnar drift of the digits.[43,44] Associated tendon rupture is usually not amenable to primary repair. Tendon grafting or end-to-side repairs are more commonly used to help restore function. The most commonly affected extensor tendons include the extensor pollicis longus (at Lister's tubercle), extensor digiti minimi (at the level of the DRUJ), and extensor digitorum comminis (**Fig. 3**).[45] Associated joint destruction and bony spurs can also be treated in conjunction with synovectomy.

Flexor Tenosynovectomy and Volar Wrist Synovectomy

Because volar wrist swelling is generally less evident than that on the dorsum, the flexor tendons in the volar wrist are vulnerable to injury. These tendons are located adjacent to the volar wrist capsule, deep to the transverse carpal ligament, and crowd into the carpal tunnel space that has little or no give. Osteophyte formations with associated joint disease in the volar wrist combine to contribute to attritional tendon rupture. The flexor pollicis longus is the most common flexor tendon to rupture, followed by the flexor digitorum profundus to the index finger.[3,46]

Unfortunately, tendon irritation and pending rupture may be clinically subtle, and is compounded by the fact that the immunosuppressive effects of antirheumatic medications can mask and subdue the pain. Any sign of pain with resisted flexion of the fingers and wrist or loss of function can be viewed as an indication for surgery. Prompt surgical treatment with synovectomy, tenosynovectomy, and/or osteophyte debridement can help minimize risk of rupture. In patients who have already gone on to rupture, prompt surgery can afford the best chance at restoration of function.

The surgical exposure to the volar wrist may be typically done through an extended approach to the carpal tunnel. The carpal tunnel is released, and the flexor tendons can be visualized within the Parona space. Extensive tenosynovitis is commonly seen, and a complete and thorough debridement can be performed through this approach. Thereafter, attention can turn to the wrist. Bony spurs and osteophytes, when present, may be debrided and synovectomy performed. Care should be taken to preserve the extrinsic ligaments to avoid further destabilization of the wrist. Except in acute cases and injuries with minimal fraying, flexor tendon ruptures are typically not amenable to primary repair. Tendon grafting or transfers are typically more appropriate for restoration of thumb flexor tendon function. Thumb interphalangeal joint arthrodesis is an alternative option for stabilizing the thumb. In cases involving index finger flexor tendon rupture, if only the flexor digitorum superficialis (FDS) is injured and flexor digitorum profundus (FDP) is spared, no treatment is usually necessary because the FDP will likely preserve appropriate index finger function. However, if the FDP is ruptured, surgical treatment

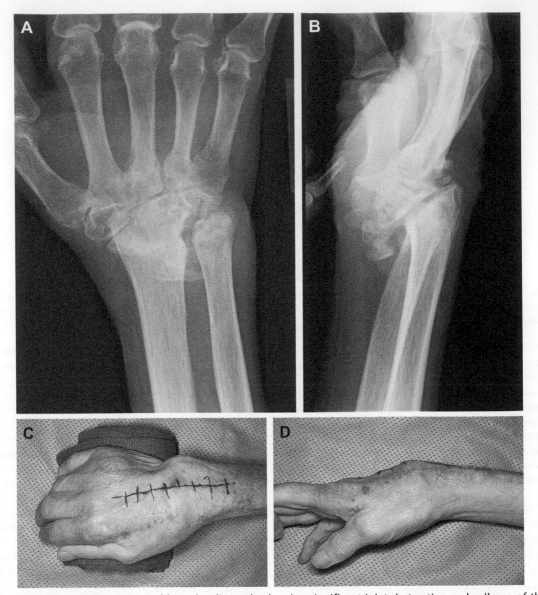

Fig. 3. (*A, B*) Anteroposterior and lateral radiographs showing significant joint destruction and collapse of the wrist with spurring of the dorsal distal radius acting as a tendon irritant. (*C, D*) Photographs of the wrist show volar translation at the wrist. (*E*) The extensor pollicis longus had ruptured and scarred in at the level of the radiocarpal joint as had the extensor digitorum comminis to the index and the extensor indicis proprius. (*F*) In addition, the extensor digiti minimi was ruptured and also scarred in ulnarly. (*G*) Spurring of the ulnar head is noted. Following tendon reconstructions, the patient underwent arthrodesis of the wrist and distal ulna resection.

is advised. Options include tendon transfer or grafting. An alternative includes distal interphalangeal joint arthrodesis in patients with an intact FDP.

TREATMENT OF DISTAL RADIOULNAR JOINT IN RHEUMATOID ARTHRITIS

Rheumatoid arthritis can affect the DRUJ, causing instability and dorsal subluxation of the distal ulna.

Supination of the carpus further exaggerates the dorsal prominence of the ulna. Pain, instability, and potential threat of tendon rupture are important considerations for surgery. Rarely is synovectomy alone an appropriate treatment. Likewise, ligament stabilization procedures such as extensor retinaculum transfer (Hubert procedure) are restricted to patients with healthy cartilage or excellent control of their inflammation. Practically

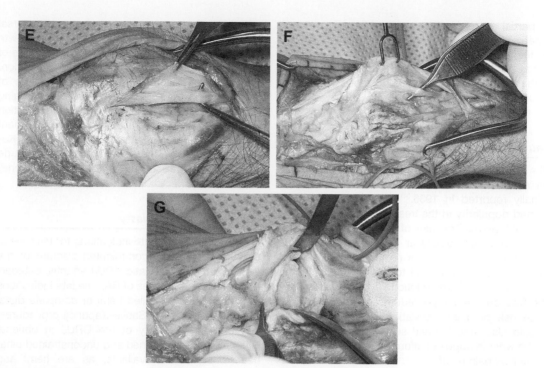

Fig. 3. (*continued*)

speaking, most treatment is directed at the arthritic joint. In these cases 3 options are commonly used: (1) distal ulna resection (Darrach procedure), (2) DRUJ arthrodesis (Sauvé-Kapanji procedure), or (3) ulna head arthroplasty.

Distal Ulna Resection (Darrach Procedure)

Initially described by Darrach in 1912, the distal ulna resection is an established treatment for arthritis of the DRUJ. The surgical approach is generally straightforward and, when appropriately performed, can generally yield reliable results. Indications include refractory DRUJ synovitis with concomitant arthritis, associated ulnar extensor tendon rupture, and caput ulna syndrome with arthritis. The procedure may also be done in patients with arthritis and ulnocarpal impingement, in association with radiocarpal arthrodesis, total wrist arthrodesis, or arthroplasty. Contraindications include patients with excessive carpal supination or at risk of ulnar translation of the carpus following distal ulna resection. In these cases, radiocarpal stabilization (eg, limited or complete wrist arthrodesis) is necessary in conjunction with the distal ulna resection.

The surgical approach for the Darrach procedure can generally be done using a dorsal exposure through the fifth dorsal compartment. Deep to the fifth compartment the capsule of the DRUJ can be incised and elevated, preserving the ECU subsheath. The joint is exposed and the head of the ulna is removed such that there is no longer an articulation with the sigmoid notch. Oblique and straight cuts have been described, but care should be taken to take the minimum amount of distal ulna. Smoothing the edges of the bone cuts helps avoid irritating the superficial soft tissues. Stabilization of the stump is also important; this can commonly be done with the distal aspect of the pronator quadratus and tightening of the dorsal capsule, using a slip of the extensor carpi ulnaris or flexor carpi ulnaris tendon.

Several reports of good outcomes regarding pain and forearm rotation following distal ulna resection have been described.[37,47] Tulipan and colleagues[48] also described good outcomes, but stressed the importance of good technique to achieve desired results. Others have reiterated this and stressed the importance of ulnar stump stabilization.[49] Unfortunately, some studies have demonstrated significant failure rates with few options for salvage.[50] Common complications include ulnar drift of the carpus, convergence of the distal ulna stump, and instability of the distal ulna.[51–54] Ishikawa and colleagues[37] recommended the Darrach procedure be performed in conjunction with wrist extensor tendon transfer or partial radiocarpal fusion to reduce the risk of ulnar carpal drift. Weakness resulting from loss of the ulnar support structures can occur, and tends to be more noticeable in patients with higher-demand lifestyles, such as those with post-traumatic arthritis or osteoarthritis, and less so in RA patients.[55]

Sauvé-Kapandji Procedure

The Sauvé-Kapandji procedure was proposed as an alternative to distal ulna resection and was initially reported in 1936.[56] This procedure has gained popularity in the treatment of RA over the past 20 years. The aim of the procedure is to create a distal radioulnar arthrodesis between the ulnar head and distal radius. A segment of ulna is removed proximal to the arthrodesis site to allow for forearm rotation. When successful, the Sauvé-Kapandji procedure should help minimize risk of ulnar translation of the carpus. It should also stabilize and support the ulnar side of the wrist in hopes of affording superior function as well as pain relief.

The procedure may be performed through the same longitudinal incision used for synovectomy or distal ulnar resection. Following exposure of the DRUJ, the cartilage from the ulnar head and sigmoid notch are denuded and provisional fixation is used. The ulnar head is positioned at the level of the radius (neutral variance) or just proximal to prevent ulnocarpal impingement. Compression screws (usually 2–3 screws) may be used to facilitate stabilization of the ulna and radius. A segment of ulna, usually 8 to 10 mm in length, can then be removed proximal to the arthrodesis site. Typically a minimum of 1 cm of ulnar resection is used to minimize chance of bony overgrowth. Multiple stabilization methods for the proximal ulnar stump have been suggested, including tenodesis with the ECU and/or flexor carpi ulnaris.[57,58] Although the success is questioned, interposition of the pronator quadratus at the ulnar gap can also be performed to stabilize the proximal stump and reduce the incidence of regrowth.

Multiple investigators have reported excellent outcomes with the Sauvé-Kapandji procedure,[59,60] but other reports suggest that there is little or no clinical or radiographic superiority over resection of the distal ulna.[61,62] Like the Darrach procedure, it is possible to resect too much ulna, resulting in proximal stump instability. Daecke and colleagues[63] suggested that situating the proximal stump less than 35 mm from the distal aspect of the radioulnar arthrodesis is associated with greater stability of the stump. Additional complications include impingement or convergence of the proximal ulnar stump

with the radius, nonunion of the fusion site, dorsal sensory branch of the ulnar nerve irritation, regrowth of the ulna, and tendon rupture. Overall, reports of complication are fewer than for distal ulna resection. However, most surgeons agree that salvage of a failed Sauvé-Kapandji can be more challenging that of a failed Darrach. Soft-tissue stabilization and custom ulnar head arthroplasty are treatment options for the painful and/or unstable Sauvé-Kapandji.[64,65] Less desirable alternatives include further proximal resection of the ulna and a one-bone forearm.[66,67]

Ulnar Head Arthroplasty

The acute or immediate indications for ulnar head arthroplasty include comminuted fracture of the distal ulna, posttraumatic DRUJ arthritis, osteoarthritis, and select cases of RA. The late indications include salvage for failed hemi or complete distal ulna resection, failed Sauvé-Kapandji procedures, and chronic instability of the DRUJ in patients with arthritis. Constrained and unconstrained ulnar head designs are available, as are hemi and complete DRUJ arthroplasty systems. In addition, a hemi-head and complete ulnar head replacements are available. At this time, the unconstrained hemi-arthroplasty is the most commonly used. The advantage of a successful ulnar head arthroplasty includes improved stability of the forearm axis, elimination of convergence, and improved function when compared with ulnar head resection. Contraindications include advanced destruction and uncorrectable instability of the DRUJ, uncorrected malunion of the distal radius, skeletal immaturity, prior infection, and known sensitivity or allergy to implant materials.

The surgical approach to the DRUJ can be similar to those of the distal ulna resection and Sauvé-Kapandji. Care should be taken to tag and protect the soft-tissue stabilizers including the dorsal radioulnar ligaments, the ECU and its subsheath, and the dorsal capsule. These structures are essential in helping stabilize the implant. In cases of hemi-arthroplasty, the amount of ulna head removed is based on a cutting guide. The ulnar canal is broached and the trial stem can be inserted. Implant size can be based on the resected native ulnar head. Trialing of the ulnar head will assist in confirming appropriate length and stability. Following implant placement, the soft tissues are reapproximated for stability. Some implants have holes or slots for sutures to aid in stabilizing the implant. If there is a soft-tissue defect causing instability, the flexor carpi ulnaris tendon (Linscheid-Hue procedure), free palmaris longus graft (Adams-Berger procedure), or rerouting of the brachioradialis may be used for reconstruction.

Preliminary outcomes with the ulnar head arthroplasty for the treatment of arthrosis and instability have been encouraging.[68,69] However, the numbers are few and longer follow-up will better validate its use for the treatment of RA. Most surgeons stress the importance of soft-tissue stabilization to ensure success of this procedure by using local tissues such as ECU subsheath, triangular fibrocartilage complex, and dorsal-volar capsule. However, many patients with long-standing RA, poorly controlled inflammation, and instability of the DRUJ may be considered poor candidates for ulnar head arthroplasty.

RADIOCARPAL AND PAN-CARPAL ARTHRITIS

Disease of the radiocarpal and midcarpal joints is common in patients with RA. Surgical treatment options for these diseases include partial or complete wrist arthrodesis and total wrist arthroplasty.

Partial Wrist Arthrodesis

The indications of partial wrist fusion include patients with disease primarily localized to the radiocarpal joint while sparing the midcarpal joint, progressive ulnar translation of the carpus, palmar subluxation of the wrist, and radiocarpal instability. In addition, it may be used in association with distal ulna resection to obviate the risk of ulnar carpal drift. The most commonly used partial wrist arthrodesis procedures include radiolunate arthrodesis and radioscapholunate arthrodesis. Contraindications include midcarpal arthrosis or rapidly progressive inflammatory process. The obvious advantage of partial wrist arthrodesis is that it preserves some range of motion in the wrist.

The procedure can be performed through a standard dorsal approach to the wrist. The wrist may be exposed through a ligament-sparing approach and synovectomy is performed at the same time. On exposure of the radiocarpal joint, the remaining cartilage is denuded and bone ends approximated. It is important to reduce the lunate to a neutral position for fusion. Extension of the lunate will limit wrist flexion. Abrupt overcorrection of the carpal height has also been shown to accelerate the arthritic process at the mid-carpal joint, especially in patients with long-standing preoperative deformity and collapse.[70] Stabilization of the arthrodesis may be performed with k-wires **(Fig. 4)**, plates and screws, compression screws, tension bands, or staples.[71–74] Bone grafting is recommended for interposition at the fusion site and may be harvested from the distal radius,

proximal ulna, distal ulna (in cases of distal ulna resection), or iliac crest.

Outcomes for partial wrist arthrodesis are generally reliable.[11,70,73,74] Outcomes for the prevention of ulnar drift in patients who undergo ulnar head resection have also been favorable.[71,72,75] Complications include nonunion, malunion, progression of mid-carpal arthritis, tendon irritation/rupture, and painful hardware. Nonunion is uncommon. The presence of mid-carpal arthritis has been shown in some studies to not be an absolute contraindication to partial wrist fusion.[11,76] In addition, the progression of mid-carpal arthritis following partial wrist fusion appears generally well tolerated.[70]

Total Wrist Arthrodesis

For more diffuse or advanced wrist disease, total wrist arthrodesis is an appropriate treatment option. It is indicated for patients with pan-carpal disease, pain, severe deformity, and poor soft-tissue support. Arthrodesis does significantly limit wrist motion, and it is important for the patient to understand the limitations associated with this procedure. One can get a good sense of an arthrodesis by wearing a wrist splint preoperatively for a period of time. The ideal position of fusion for each individual needs to be discussed preoperatively.

The technique typically involves a longitudinal approach to the dorsal wrist. The retinaculum is released between the third and fourth compartments. The carpus may be exposed through a distally based flap, and H-shaped or T-shaped capsulotomy. Following synovectomy, the bone ends are denuded in preparation for arthrodesis. The minimum number of joints included in a total wrist arthrodesis includes radiolunate, radioscaphoid, scaphocapitate, capitolunate, and capitometacarpal joints. The ideal position of fusion is slight extension and ulnar deviation.[77] By contrast, some surgeons prefer fusion in the neutral position, arguing that it allows for easier pronosupination and better balancing of the flexor and extensor tendons.[78] However, the position can be customized based on hand dominance and function of the contralateral wrist. In cases of bilateral disease, one should fuse the dominant side in a limited extension and the nondominant side in neutral (or slight flexion) to complement each side and maximize function. Five degrees of flexion to 30° of extension appears to be well tolerated. Supplemental bone graft should be harvested from the iliac crest or distal radius or ulna (when resected). Dorsal wrist fusion plates are commonly used, and are designed to provide a preferred position of moderate extension and

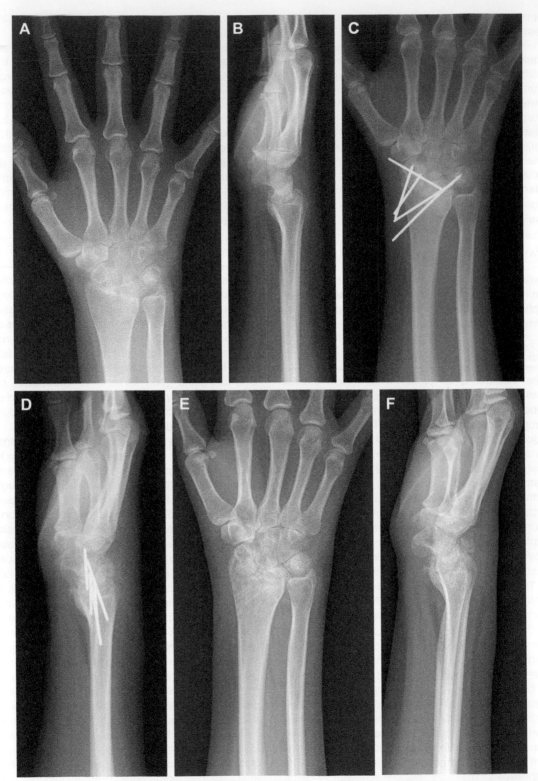

Fig. 4. (*A, B*) An anteroposterior and lateral radiograph of a 33-year-old woman with RA primarily causing joint destruction of the radiocarpal joint. (*B, C*) The patient underwent radioscapholunate arthrodesis with k-wire stabilization. The distal radioulnar joint was minimally affected by her disease and was preserved. She maintained a functional arc of motion, and (*D–F*) show her radiographs following pin removal.

ulnar deviation of the wrist. However, in patients with advanced osteoporosis, thin skin, and subcutaneous tissues, Steinmann pins, k-wires, and tension band can also be used. Preservation of the volar lip of the distal radius will help maintain the tension and length of the wrist and preserve the integrity of the carpal tunnel.

Most published outcomes of total wrist arthrodesis show that it is safe and reliable.[78,79] Meads and colleagues[80] reported excellent results of wrist arthrodesis with precontoured Synthes (Paoli, PA, USA) dorsal fusion plates (**Fig. 5**). Intramedullary Steinmann pins have also been shown to provide excellent clinical outcomes.[81,82] A comparison study of fusion plates versus intramedullary fixation has shown that both provide excellent fusion rates; however, complications tended to be higher in the intramedullary pin fixation group, and plates provided a superior position of the wrist.[83,84] Another comparison between plate fixation and the Mannerfelt technique demonstrated similar reduction in pain and functional improvement between groups.[77] Complications of wrist fusions include nonunion (especially of the carpometacarpal joint), painful hardware, hardware failure, tendon irritation, and limited range of motion in the finger. In an effort to reconcile some of the difficulties with the third carpometacarpal joint nonunion, some surgeons have advocated not trying to fuse the carpometacarpal joint, and planning a hardware

removal on successful radiocarpal and midcarpal fusion.

Total Wrist Arthroplasty

Generally considered a higher-risk, higher-reward procedure, total wrist arthroplasty is an alternative to arthrodesis. The primary advantage is preservation of wrist motion. The primary disadvantage lies in the durability and reliability of the prosthesis. Early designs were hinged silicone implants. Cemented and cementless unconstrained designs gained popularity in the 1970s and 1980s. Although these implants had superior material properties compared with silicone, the failure rates were substantial and revision rates of 20% at 5 years have been reported.[85] Most failures were secondary to problems at the distal (carpal) component, although imbalance and dislocation were also problems.[86-89] The most recent designs use screw fixation into the carpus to improve the distal component durability and minimal resection of the distal radius. The newer designs also have more physiologic wrist kinematics and essentially function more like a surface replacement. Minimal bone resection affords preservation of the volar and dorsal supporting structures, as well as better maintenance of the wrist length and tension, which allows for better soft-tissue balancing and muscle-tendon mechanics. Because these newer designs

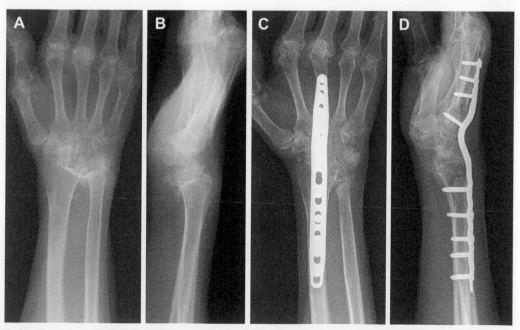

Fig. 5. (A, B) Anteroposterior and lateral radiographs of a 58-year-old woman with extensive pan-carpal, radiocarpal, and distal radioulnar joint RA. (C, D) Anteroposterior and lateral radiographs show healed fusion and stable distal ulna resection. The patient had excellent pain relief and functional improvement after healing.

essentially "resurface" the radial side of the joint, it is not always necessary to remove the ulnar head, and ulnar head arthroplasty can be performed simultaneously. Because they are more precise, these total wrist arthroplasty designs are technically more demanding, and require precise positioning and alignment of the total wrist components. It is thought by some investigators that these newer designs may expand the indications for total wrist arthroplasty beyond patients with inflammatory arthritis and RA to include scapholunate advanced collapse, scaphoid nonunion advanced collapse, primary osteoarthritis, and failed partial wrist fusions. Further studies will help to better validate these implants and better define their role in the management of wrist arthritis.

The procedure is performed through a dorsal approach to the wrist. The wrist is exposed in a similar fashion to that for wrist arthrodesis. Capsular flaps are preserved. Appropriate centering of the implant is critical to ensure correct placement and alignment. The head of the capitate is felt to be the keystone to centering the prosthesis. Cuts are made to preserve the kinematics of the wrist while resecting the minimal amount of bone. The radial component is usually prepared first. The distal component is then prepared. The use of fluoroscopy helps to confirm appropriate alignment, broaching, and implant placement. Screws help to secure the distal component, and the radial component is press-fit. Most surgeons prefer to avoid the use of cement because it

makes revision or salvage more challenging. With minimal bone resection, the new total wrist generally provides excellent carpal stability (**Fig. 6**).

Studies have demonstrated that when successful, patients prefer arthroplasty to arthrodesis primarily because of improved ease of activities of daily living and hygiene.[90,91] Cost-utility analysis suggests that arthroplasty and arthrodesis are cost-effective and that total wrist arthroplasty is only minimally more costly than arthrodesis.[92] The investigators concluded that arthroplasty is worth considering and is not as cost-prohibitive as previously thought. In addition, surgeons and rheumatologists believe that arthroplasty was associated with the highest expected improvement in quality of life, but it appears they were not convinced that arthroplasty is superior (at least not at this time).[93,94]

Early follow-up studies of total wrist arthroplasty have shown that the outcomes and patient satisfaction are encouraging.[95] In a longer follow-up study, Strunk and Bracker[96] reviewed 41 implants (10 of which were newer generation) in 36 patients with an average 5.3-year follow-up. Failure rates were approximately 15% and all but 6 patients were satisfied or very satisfied, while all but one had improved pain. The investigators conceded that total wrist arthroplasty carries a higher risk than arthrodesis, and concluded that results are dependent on careful patient selection. Further and longer-term studies will better define the role of arthroplasty in the management of wrist RA.

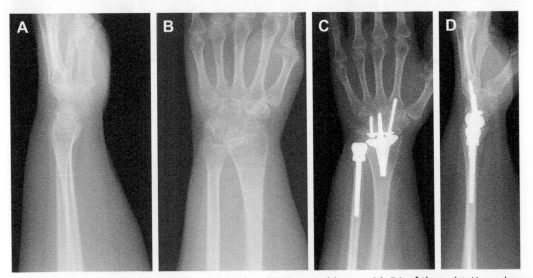

Fig. 6. (A, B) Anteroposterior and lateral radiographs of a 55-year-old man with RA of the wrist. He underwent total wrist arthroplasty with concomitant ulnar head arthroplasty. (C, D) Anteroposterior and lateral radiographs at 2 years after surgery demonstrate stable arthroplasties and excellent alignment of the wrist.

SUMMARY

The wrist is commonly affected in patients with RA. Pharmacologic agents including anti-TNF medications have shown promise in ameliorating the inflammatory-mediated destruction of the joints and decreasing the need for surgical intervention. Surgical treatment options are varied and are based on the degree of joint destruction and synovitis. Tendon ruptures are not uncommon and, pending rupture or frank injury, require early surgical intervention. The DRUJ is commonly affected, and surgical treatment options include distal ulna resection, the Sauvé-Kapandji procedure (distal radioulnar joint fusion), and ulnar head arthroplasty. For more advanced radiocarpal or midcarpal disease, partial or complete wrist arthrodesis and wrist arthroplasty are appropriate treatments.

REFERENCES

1. Crilly A, Maiden N, Capell HA, et al. Genotyping for disease associated HLA DR beta 1 alleles and the need for early joint surgery in rheumatoid arthritis: a quantitative evaluation. Ann Rheum Dis 1999;58: 114–7.
2. Trieb K. Treatment of the wrist in rheumatoid arthritis. J Hand Surg Am 2008;33:113–23.
3. Mannerfelt L, Norman O. Attrition ruptures of flexor tendons in rheumatoid arthritis caused by bony spurs in the carpal tunnel. A Clinical and Radiological Study. J Bone Joint Surg Br 1969;51:270–7.
4. Vaughan-Jackson OJ. Rupture of extensor tendons by attrition at the inferior radio-ulnar joint; report of two cases. J Bone Joint Surg Br 1948;30:528–30.
5. Backdahl M. The caput ulnae syndrome in rheumatoid arthritis. A study of the morphology, abnormal anatomy and clinical picture. Acta Rheumatol Scand Suppl 1963;5:1–75.
6. Stack HG, Vaughan-Jackson OJ. The zig-zag deformity in the rheumatoid hand. Hand 1971;3:62–7.
7. Wilson RL, DeVito MC. Extensor tendon problems in rheumatoid arthritis. Hand Clin 1996;12:551–9.
8. Shinoda J, Hashizume H, McCown C, et al. Carpal tunnel syndrome grading system in rheumatoid arthritis. J Orthop Sci 2002;7:188–93.
9. Bywaters EG. The early radiological signs of rheumatoid arthritis. Bull Rheum Dis 1960;11:231–4.
10. Martel W, Hayes JT, Duff IF. The pattern of bone erosion in the hand and wrist in rheumatoid arthritis. Radiology 1965;84:204–14.
11. Taleisnik J. Combined radiocarpal arthrodesis and midcarpal (lunocapitate) arthroplasty for treatment of rheumatoid arthritis of the wrist. J Hand Surg Am 1987;12:1–8.
12. Hindley CJ, Stanley JK. The rheumatoid wrist: patterns of disease progression. A review of 50 wrists. J Hand Surg Br 1991;16:275–9.
13. Hodgson SP, Stanley JK, Muirhead A. The Wrightington classification of rheumatoid wrist X-rays: a guide to surgical management. J Hand Surg Br 1989;14:451–5.
14. Larsen A, Dale K, Eek M. Radiographic evaluation of rheumatoid arthritis and related conditions by standard reference films. Acta Radiol Diagn (Stockh) 1977;18:481–91.
15. Simmen BR, Huber H. [The wrist joint in chronic polyarthritis—a new classification based on the type of destruction in relation to the natural course and the consequences for surgical therapy]. Handchir Mikrochir Plast Chir 1994;26:182–9 [in German].
16. Lisbona MP, Maymo J, Perich J, et al. Rapid reduction in tenosynovitis of the wrist and fingers evaluated by MRI in patients with rheumatoid arthritis after treatment with etanercept. Ann Rheum Dis 2010;69:1117–22.
17. McQueen F, Clarke A, McHaffie A, et al. Assessment of cartilage loss at the wrist in rheumatoid arthritis using a new MRI scoring system. Ann Rheum Dis 2010;69. [Epub ahead of print].
18. Haavardsholm EA, Boyesen P, Ostergaard M, et al. Magnetic resonance imaging findings in 84 patients with early rheumatoid arthritis: bone marrow oedema predicts erosive progression. Ann Rheum Dis 2008; 67:794–800.
19. Egan M, Brosseau L, Farmer M, et al. Splints/orthoses in the treatment of rheumatoid arthritis. Cochrane Database Syst Rev 2003;1:CD004018.
20. Veehof MM, Taal E, Heijnsdijk-Rouwenhorst LM, et al. Efficacy of wrist working splints in patients with rheumatoid arthritis: a randomized controlled study. Arthritis Rheum 2008;59:1698–704.
21. Adams J, Burridge J, Mullee M, et al. The clinical effectiveness of static resting splints in early rheumatoid arthritis: a randomized controlled trial. Rheumatology (Oxford) 2008;47:1548–53.
22. Lopes RV, Furtado RN, Parmigiani L, et al. Accuracy of intra-articular injections in peripheral joints performed blindly in patients with rheumatoid arthritis. Rheumatology (Oxford) 2008;47:1792–4.
23. Konai MS, Vilar Furtado RN, Dos Santos MF, et al. Monoarticular corticosteroid injection versus systemic administration in the treatment of rheumatoid arthritis patients: a randomized double-blind controlled study. Clin Exp Rheumatol 2009;27: 214–21.
24. Weitoft T, Ronnblom L. Randomised controlled study of postinjection immobilisation after intra-articular glucocorticoid treatment for wrist synovitis. Ann Rheum Dis 2003;62:1013–5.
25. Bliddal H, Terslev L, Qvistgaard E, et al. Safety of intra-articular injection of etanercept in small-joint

arthritis: an uncontrolled, pilot-study with independent imaging assessment. Joint Bone Spine 2006;73: 714–7.

26. Bliddal H, Terslev L, Qvistgaard E, et al. A randomized, controlled study of a single intra-articular injection of etanercept or glucocorticosteroids in patients with rheumatoid arthritis. Scand J Rheumatol 2006;35:341–5.

27. James D, Young A, Kulinskaya E, et al. Orthopaedic intervention in early rheumatoid arthritis. Occurrence and predictive factors in an inception cohort of 1064 patients followed for 5 years. Rheumatology (Oxford) 2004;43:369–76.

28. Jain A, Witbreuk M, Ball C, et al. Influence of steroids and methotrexate on wound complications after elective rheumatoid hand and wrist surgery. J Hand Surg Am 2002;27:449–55.

29. Favalli EG, Desiati F, Atzeni F, et al. Serious infections during anti-TNFalpha treatment in rheumatoid arthritis patients. Autoimmun Rev 2009;8: 266–73.

30. Marchal L, D'Haens G, Van Assche G, et al. The risk of post-operative complications associated with infliximab therapy for Crohn's disease: a controlled cohort study. Aliment Pharmacol Ther 2004;19:749–54.

31. Alderman AK, Chung KC, Kim HM, et al. Effectiveness of rheumatoid hand surgery: contrasting perceptions of hand surgeons and rheumatologists. J Hand Surg Am 2003;28:3–11 [discussion: 12–3].

32. Millender LH, Nalebuff EA. Preventive surgery—tenosynovectomy and synovectomy. Orthop Clin North Am 1975;6:765–92.

33. Ryu J, Saito S, Honda T, et al. Risk factors and prophylactic tenosynovectomy for extensor tendon ruptures in the rheumatoid hand. J Hand Surg Br 1998;23:658–61.

34. Mannerfelt L. On surgery of the rheumatoid hand: consensus and controversy. J Hand Surg Br 1989; 14:259–60.

35. Shapiro JS. The wrist in rheumatoid arthritis. Hand Clin 1996;12:477–98.

36. Brumfield R Jr, Kuschner SH, Gellman H, et al. Results of dorsal wrist synovectomies in the rheumatoid hand. J Hand Surg Am 1990;15:733–5.

37. Ishikawa H, Hanyu T, Tajima T. Rheumatoid wrists treated with synovectomy of the extensor tendons and the wrist joint combined with a Darrach procedure. J Hand Surg Am 1992;17:1109–17.

38. Thirupathi RG, Ferlic DC, Clayton ML. Dorsal wrist synovectomy in rheumatoid arthritis—a long-term study. J Hand Surg Am 1983;8:848–56.

39. Adolfsson L, Frisen M. Arthroscopic synovectomy of the rheumatoid wrist. A 3.8 year follow-up. J Hand Surg Br 1997;22:711–3.

40. Park MJ, Ahn JH, Kang JS. Arthroscopic synovectomy of the wrist in rheumatoid arthritis. J Bone Joint Surg Br 2003;85:1011–5.

41. Nakamura H, Nagashima M, Ishigami S, et al. The anti-rheumatic effect of multiple synovectomy in patients with refractory rheumatoid arthritis. Int Orthop 2000;24:242–5.

42. Ochi T, Iwase R, Kimura T, et al. Effect of early synovectomy on the course of rheumatoid arthritis. J Rheumatol 1991;18:1794–8.

43. Clayton ML, Ferlic DC. Tendon transfer for radial rotation of the wrist in rheumatoid arthritis. Clin Orthop Relat Res 1974;100:176–85.

44. Ito J, Koshino T, Okamoto R, et al. Radiologic evaluation of the rheumatoid hand after synovectomy and extensor carpi radialis longus transfer to extensor carpi ulnaris. J Hand Surg Am 2003;28:585–90.

45. Norris SH. Surgery for the rheumatoid wrist and hand. Ann Rheum Dis 1990;49(Suppl 2):863–70.

46. Ertel AN, Millender LH, Nalebuff E, et al. Flexor tendon ruptures in patients with rheumatoid arthritis. J Hand Surg Am 1988;13:860–6.

47. Jensen CM. Synovectomy with resection of the distal ulna in rheumatoid arthritis of the wrist. Acta Orthop Scand 1983;54:754–9.

48. Tulipan DJ, Eaton RG, Eberhart RE. The Darrach procedure defended: technique redefined and long-term follow-up. J Hand Surg Am 1991;16: 438–44.

49. Syed AA, Lam WL, Agarwal M, et al. Stabilization of the ulna stump after Darrach's procedure at the wrist. Int Orthop 2003;27:235–9.

50. Bieber EJ, Linscheid RL, Dobyns JH, et al. Failed distal ulna resections. J Hand Surg Am 1988;13: 193–200.

51. Field J, Majkowski RJ, Leslie IJ. Poor results of Darrach's procedure after wrist injuries. J Bone Joint Surg Br 1993;75:53–7.

52. Jain A, Ball C, Nanchahal J. Functional outcome following extensor synovectomy and excision of the distal ulna in patients with rheumatoid arthritis. J Hand Surg Br 2003;28:531–6.

53. McKee MD, Richards RR. Dynamic radio-ulnar convergence after the Darrach procedure. J Bone Joint Surg Br 1996;78:413–8.

54. Van Gemert AM, Spauwen PH. Radiological evaluation of the long-term effects of resection of the distal ulna in rheumatoid arthritis. J Hand Surg Br 1994;19: 330–3.

55. Fraser KE, Diao E, Peimer CA, et al. Comparative results of resection of the distal ulna in rheumatoid arthritis and post-traumatic conditions. J Hand Surg Br 1999;24:667–70.

56. Sauve L, Kapandji M. Nouvelle technique de traitement chirurgical des luxations recidivantes isolees de l'extremiite inferirure du cubitus. J Chir 1936;47: 589–94.

57. Lamey DM, Fernandez DL. Results of the modified Sauvé-Kapandji procedure in the treatment of chronic posttraumatic derangement of the distal

radioulnar joint. J Bone Joint Surg Am 1998;80: 1758–69.

58. Minami A, Iwasaki N, Ishikawa J, et al. Stabilization of the proximal ulnar stump in the Sauvé-Kapandji procedure by using the extensor carpi ulnaris tendon: long-term follow-up studies. J Hand Surg Am 2006;31:440–4.

59. Fujita S, Masada K, Takeuchi E, et al. Modified Sauvé-Kapandji procedure for disorders of the distal radioulnar joint in patients with rheumatoid arthritis. J Bone Joint Surg Am 2005;87:134–9.

60. Vincent KA, Szabo RM, Agee JM. The Sauvé-Kapandji procedure for reconstruction of the rheumatoid distal radioulnar joint. J Hand Surg Am 1993; 18:978–83.

61. George MS, Kiefhaber TR, Stern PJ. The Sauvé-Kapandji procedure and the Darrach procedure for distal radio-ulnar joint dysfunction after Colles' fracture. J Hand Surg Br 2004;29:608–13.

62. Kobayashi A, Futami T, Tadano I, et al. Radiographic comparative evaluation of the Sauvé-Kapandji procedure and the Darrach procedure for rheumatoid wrist reconstruction. Mod Rheumatol 2005;15: 187–90.

63. Daecke W, Martini AK, Schneider S, et al. Amount of ulnar resection is a predictive factor for ulnar instability problems after the Sauvé-Kapandji procedure: a retrospective study of 44 patients followed for 1–13 years. Acta Orthop 2006;77:290–7.

64. Fernandez DL, Joneschild ES, Abella DM. Treatment of failed Sauvé-Kapandji procedures with a spherical ulnar head prosthesis. Clin Orthop Relat Res 2006; 445:100–7.

65. Scheker LR. Implant arthroplasty for the distal radioulnar joint. J Hand Surg Am 2008;33:1639–44.

66. Peterson CA 2nd, Maki S, Wood MB. Clinical results of the one-bone forearm. J Hand Surg Am 1995;20: 609–18.

67. Wolfe SW, Mih AD, Hotchkiss RN, et al. Wide excision of the distal ulna: a multicenter case study. J Hand Surg Am 1998;23:222–8.

68. Willis AA, Berger RA, Cooney WP 3rd. Arthroplasty of the distal radioulnar joint using a new ulnar head endoprosthesis: preliminary report. J Hand Surg Am 2007;32:177–89.

69. Vs J, Herbert TJ, Fernandez DL, et al. [Ulnar head prosthesis]. Orthopade 2003;32:809–15 [in German].

70. Borisch N, Haussmann P. Radiolunate arthrodesis in the rheumatoid wrist: a retrospective clinical and radiological longterm follow-up. J Hand Surg Br 2002;27:61–72.

71. Doets HC, Raven EE. A procedure for stabilising and preserving mobility in the arthritic wrist. J Bone Joint Surg Br 1999;81:1013–6.

72. Linscheid RL, Dobyns JH. Radiolunate arthrodesis. J Hand Surg Am 1985;10:821–9.

73. Stanley JK, Boot DA. Radio-lunate arthrodesis. J Hand Surg Br 1989;14:283–7.

74. Ishikawa H, Murasawa A, Nakazono K. Long-term follow-up study of radiocarpal arthrodesis for the rheumatoid wrist. J Hand Surg Am 2005;30:658–66.

75. Ishikawa H, Hanyu T, Saito H, et al. Limited arthrodesis for the rheumatoid wrist. J Hand Surg Am 1992; 17:1103–9.

76. Della Santa D, Chamay A. Radiological evolution of the rheumatoid wrist after radio-lunate arthrodesis. J Hand Surg Br 1995;20:146–54.

77. Toma CD, Machacek P, Bitzan P, et al. Fusion of the wrist in rheumatoid arthritis: a clinical and functional evaluation of two surgical techniques. J Bone Joint Surg Br 2007;89:1620–6.

78. Clayton ML, Ferlic DC. Arthrodesis of the arthritic wrist. Clin Orthop 1984;187:89–93.

79. Mannerfelt L, Malmsten M. Arthrodesis of the wrist in rheumatoid arthritis: a technique without external fixation. Scand J Plast Reconstr Surg 1971;5:124–30.

80. Meads BM, Scougall PJ, Hargreaves IC. Wrist arthrodesis using a Synthes wrist fusion plate. J Hand Surg Br 2003;28:571–4.

81. Barbier O, Saels P, Rombouts JJ, et al. Long-term functional results of wrist arthrodesis in rheumatoid arthritis. J Hand Surg Br 1999;24:27–31.

82. Lee DH, Carroll RE. Wrist arthrodesis: a combined intramedullary pin and autogenous iliac crest bone graft technique. J Hand Surg Am 1994;19:733–40.

83. Howard AC, Stanley D, Getty CJ. Wrist arthrodesis in rheumatoid arthritis. A comparison of two methods of fusion. J Hand Surg Br 1993;18:377–80.

84. Rehak DC, Kasper P, Baratz ME, et al. A comparison of plate and pin fixation for arthrodesis of the rheumatoid wrist. Orthopedics 2000;23:43–8.

85. Cobb TK, Beckenbaugh RD. Biaxial total-wrist arthroplasty. J Hand Surg Am 1996;21:1011–21.

86. Figgie HE 3rd, Ranawat CS, Inglis AE, et al. Preliminary results of total wrist arthroplasty in rheumatoid arthritis using the trispherical total wrist arthroplasty. J Arthroplasty 1988;3:9–15.

87. Meuli HC. Meuli total wrist arthroplasty. Clin Orthop Relat Res 1984;187:107–11.

88. Takwale VJ, Nuttall D, Trail IA, et al. Biaxial total wrist replacement in patients with rheumatoid arthritis. Clinical review, survivorship and radiological analysis. J Bone Joint Surg Br 2002;84:692–9.

89. Volz RG. Total wrist arthroplasty—a new surgical procedure. ONA J 1977;4:86–8.

90. Vicar AJ, Burton RI. Surgical management of the rheumatoid wrist—fusion or arthroplasty. J Hand Surg Am 1986;11:790–7.

91. Murphy DM, Khoury JG, Imbriglia JE, et al. Comparison of arthroplasty and arthrodesis for the rheumatoid wrist. J Hand Surg Am 2003;28:570–6.

92. Cavaliere CM, Chung KC. A cost-utility analysis of nonsurgical management, total wrist arthroplasty,

and total wrist arthrodesis in rheumatoid arthritis. J Hand Surg Am 2010;35:379–91, e372.

93. Cavaliere CM, Chung KC. Total wrist arthroplasty and total wrist arthrodesis in rheumatoid arthritis: a decision analysis from the hand surgeons' perspective. J Hand Surg Am 2008;33:1744–55, e1741–2.

94. Cavaliere CM, Oppenheimer AJ, Chung KC. Reconstructing the rheumatoid wrist: a utility analysis comparing total wrist fusion and total wrist arthroplasty from the perspectives of rheumatologists and hand surgeons. Hand (N Y) 2010;5:9–18.

95. Divelbiss BJ, Sollerman C, Adams BD. Early results of the universal total wrist arthroplasty in rheumatoid arthritis. J Hand Surg Am 2002;27:195–204.

96. Strunk S, Bracker W. [Wrist joint arthroplasty: results after 41 prostheses]. Handchir Mikrochir Plast Chir 2009;41:141–7 [in German].

Rheumatoid Thumb

George S.M. Dyer, MD[a,b,*], Barry P. Simmons, MD[b]

KEYWORDS

- Rheumatoid arthritis • MCP joint • Surgical management
- Arthroplasty

The hand is the main tactile sensory organ and is uniquely designed for fine motor activities. Any deviation from the normal architecture or limitation from a painful condition may lead to disability.

It has been estimated that 50% of the "value" of the hand is from the thumb, which was defined by the American Medical Association standards for disability for the thumb.

NORMAL ANATOMY

Motion at the various joints of the thumb axis varies within the population. The sum of the thumb carpometacarpal (CMC), thumb metacarpal (MCP), and thumb interphalangeal (IP) joint motion is about 180° in most healthy people, but the proportion of motion at each joint is distributed differently because some people have stiffer CMC joints but looser MCP and IP joints, or vice versa. Physiologic hyperextension of the IP joint is important for normal function. Disease may change these proportions. Patients with arthritis of the thumb CMC joint may compensate for the loss of CMC motion by hyperextending their thumb MCP joint to preserve the span of the first web space to encompass large objects. To a lesser degree, MP joint hyperextension is physiologic.

In the coronal plane, there is minimal intrinsic bony stability in the units of the thumb. At the IP joint, there is bicondylar congruence of the distal phalanx on the proximal phalanx. However, at the MCP joint, the articulation is round-on-round, and stability is maintained entirely by the integrity of collateral ligaments. Although there is biconcave or "saddle" congruence at the CMC joint, stability depends on capsuloligamentous structures.

In the sagittal plane, the attitude of the segments of the thumb depends on the balance between the flexor and extensor tendons and the integrity of the volar plates.

CLASSIFICATION AND PATHOPHYSIOLOGY

Rheumatoid arthritis (RA) is fundamentally an inflammatory disease of the soft tissues. Deformities of the thumb arise from abnormal stretching of ligament and capsular structures, as well as from ruptures and subluxations of the tendons. The bony abnormalities and cartilage loss are generally secondary effects, resulting from the erosive properties of the inflammatory pannus.

At the early stages of disease, stopping or modifying the inflammatory process arrests the advancement of bony changes. However, once dynamic instability of the thumb has begun, it may be too late to prevent deformity and loss of function.

In 1968, Nalebuff[1] described a systematic classification scheme for understanding and treating these deformities based on the initiating pathologic event. His original classification has been expanded to include additional pathologic entities.

Type I boutonnière deformity begins with synovitis at the MP joint, which weakens the joint capsule and associated ligaments. The extensor hood becomes attenuated, which effectively stretches the extensor pollicis brevis (EPB) and allows the extensor pollicis longus (EPL) to sublux volarly and ulnarly. The IP joint becomes secondarily hyperextended as extensor power is concentrated distally. When pinch is attempted, the thumb collapses with hyperextension at the IP joint and

[a] VA Boston Healthcare, 150 South Huntington Avenue, Jamaica Plain, MA 02130, USA
[b] Hand/Upper Extremity Service, Department of Orthopaedic Surgery, Brigham and Women's Hospital, Harvard Medical School, 75 Francis Street, Boston, MA 02115, USA
* Corresponding author. Hand/Upper Extremity Service, Department of Orthopaedic Surgery, Brigham and Women's Hospital, Harvard Medical School, 75 Francis Street, Boston, MA 02115.
E-mail address: GDYER@PARTNERS.ORG

Hand Clin 27 (2011) 73–77
doi:10.1016/j.hcl.2010.10.001
0749-0712/11/$ – see front matter. Published by Elsevier Inc.

abnormal flexion at the MP joint. By definition, the MCP and IP deformities are passively correctable.

Type II is also a boutonnière deformity, but the MCP joint becomes fixed and the CMC joint is involved.

Type III describes a swan-neck beginning at the CMC joint. Synovitis at the CMC joint causes dorsal and radial subluxation at the base of the thumb unit, which adducts the distal end of the MCP. This adduction effectively narrows the first web space, limiting the size of the object that a patient can grasp. To compensate for this narrowness, the thumb hyperextends at the MP joint, which causes loss of volar plate competence. This hyperextension alters the flexor-extensor tendon balance in the rest of the thumb, resulting in flexion of the IP joint and hyperextension of the MP joint. Belt and colleagues[2] analyzed a retrospective 20-year cohort of patients with RA and found that among thumbs that developed more than 4 mm of CMC subluxation, 81% had developed a swan-neck deformity.

Type IV deformity describes the consequence of attrition of the ulnar collateral ligament of the thumb.

Type V is also a type of swan-neck deformity but begins with volar plate laxity at the MCP joint and spares the CMC joint.

Type VI results from mutilation and aggressive bone resorption. Telescoped shortening of the digits and loss of the articulations may demonstrate concentric wrinkling of the skin (opera-glass hand).

Although these valuable classifications describe the deformities, they do not necessarily lead the surgeon to surgical solutions. The surgical procedures depend not only on the deformity but also on the radiography findings.

MANAGEMENT

The first stage of management is to maximize medical therapy. Modern disease-modifying agents have truly revolutionized the management of this disease. It is therefore assumed that the following discussion concerns patients in whom these pharmacologic options have failed.

Other nonsurgical interventions by the hand surgeon depend on the degree of pain, instability, and other patient factors. Splinting and bracing may be useful to stop progression of the deformity, for example, by limiting hyperextension or hyperflexion at the MCP joint or the IP joint. A silver ring splint may be used on the thumb for this purpose.[3] A specific thumb orthosis may improve function.[4] A short opponens splint may be useful to control symptoms at the CMC joint. Injection of corticosteroids may reduce the pain of inflammation. Although an intriguing concept, the direct injection of a disease-modifying agent, such as etanercept, has not proved to be an effective therapy.[5]

SURGICAL MANAGEMENT

In a classic report, Terrono and colleagues[6] recommended different treatments of rheumatoid boutonnière thumb deformities depending on whether the deformity was passively correctable and the status of all the joints in the thumb unit. The investigators found a recurrence rate of 64% with MCP synovectomy combined with EPL rerouting procedure. They recommended MCP joint fusion when the deformity was moderate and the IP joint was spared and MCP joint arthroplasty for low-demand patients with arthritic changes in the IP and CMC joints to preserve thumb motion. They recommended fusing both the MCP joint and IP joint in advanced cases.

Although the modified Nalebuff classification system seems to suggest an appropriate therapy for each stage and type of deformity, in practice, the decision making of the hand surgeons with experience in managing RA is somewhat different. Some guidelines and lessons learned from the experience of the senior author (B.P.S) with management of the rheumatoid thumb are summarized as follows:

1. Destruction of all 3 joints, the CMC, MCP, and IP, is rare. This fact simplifies surgical planning.
2. Soft tissue reconstructions for thumb deformity are unlikely to correct the deformity adequately and do not maintain the intended correction in the long term. Therefore, although soft tissue correction may be performed in conjunction with joint procedures, they should not be performed alone. Despite the excellent categorization of deformities and suggested procedures, Dr Nalebuff ultimately abandoned pure soft tissue procedures.
3. Mobility is maintained in as many joints as possible. At the CMC joint, arthroplasty is the procedure of choice. At the MCP joint, arthroplasty or arthrodesis is the option, partly depending on the condition of the IP joint. At the IP level, arthrodesis is the usual option. It is preferable, when there is both MCP and IP disease, to not fuse both joints.

The combination of these procedures and their applications to various deformity patterns are described in the following sections.

Boutonnière Thumb

In these cases, there is flexion of the MCP joint and hyperextension or radial deviation of the IP joint. The MCP joint maybe radially deviated as well.

Radiological evaluation shows joint destruction of the MCP joint and usually destruction of the IP joint (**Fig. 1**). The procedures of choice in this combination are MCP silicone arthroplasty and IP fusion. When there is radial deviation at the MCP level, the concern is instability. However, the radial deviation is almost always because of bone loss, not incompetence of the ulnar collateral ligament. Therefore, once the deviation is corrected and the proper size prosthesis is used, the deformity is corrected.

At the IP level, if minimal destruction is seen on radiography, a terminal tendon release may be performed. Although this procedure corrects the deformity initially, in the vast majority of cases, hyperextension recurs, with subsequent increased deformity at the MCP joint. For isolated IP pain and/or deformity, so often seen in psoriatic arthritis, arthrodesis of the IP joint is the procedure of choice (**Figs. 2–4**).

Swan-Neck Thumb

In the swan-neck thumb, surgery is directed at the CMC and MCP joints. Although it is desirable to maintain as much motion as possible in all the joints, the deformity at the MCP level is usually so significant that arthrodesis is necessary.[7]

When deformity arises at the CMC joint, resection arthroplasty with tendon or allograft interposition is the procedure of choice. A ligament reconstruction-tendon interposition may be performed, less with the goal of a "suspensionplasty" than as a way of correcting the attitude of the thumb MCP. Correcting the radial and dorsal displacement of the base of the MCP corrects the adduction deformity distally. To achieve this correction, it is important to pull the base of the thumb MCP tightly against the index metacarpal as the tendon graft is sutured down.

TECHNICAL TIPS FOR MCP ARTHROPLASTY

A gentle curvili near or sinuous incision extending from the MCP to the IP joint gives ample and

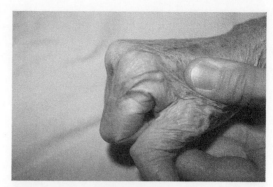
Fig. 2. Severely unstable IP joint.

flexible exposure. The interval between the EPB and EPL over the MCP joint is then incised and extended through the capsule of the MCP joint (**Figs. 5** and **6**). The overlying dorsal apparatus should be closed with the underlying capsule as a single layer at the MCP joint.

MCP arthroplasty in the thumb is different from that in the fingers. In the fingers, the ulnar collateral ligament has to be released and the extensors rebalanced. Because the thumb does not experience the sagittal band instability that is typical of the other digits, there is no need to dissect the

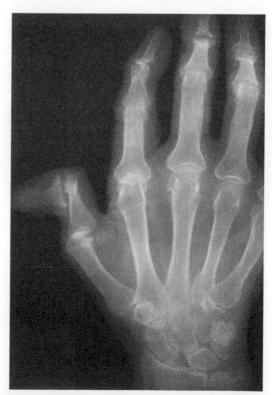
Fig. 3. Isolated IP joint destruction in psoriatic arthritis.

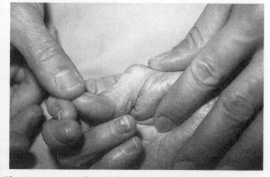
Fig. 1. Boutonnière deformity of the thumb.

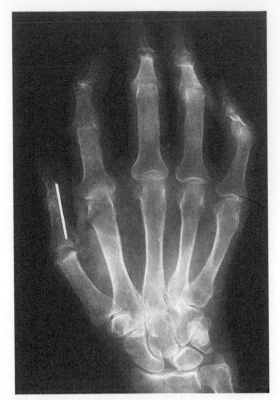

Fig. 4. IP joint fusion for IP instability.

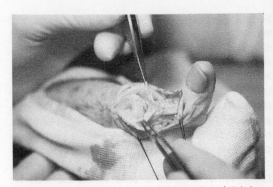

Fig. 6. Deep dorsal exposure of the MCP and IP joints.

TECHNICAL TIPS FOR IP JOINT ARTHRODESIS

The surgeon can transversely incise the terminal tendon at the IP level or continue the longitudinal incision from the MCP joint. Release of the collateral ligaments at the IP joint makes the exposure easier (**Fig. 7**).

When MCP arthroplasty is to be combined with IP joint arthrodesis, an intramedullary pin may be used, supplemented by crossed C wires. Placing the intramedullary pin first allows correction of the deformity in the radial/ulnar plane, and then rotation can be addressed. If the intramedullary pin affects the placement of the MCP silicone prosthesis, the fusion should be completed before the prosthesis is inserted. However, both joints should be prepared for the final procedure before the implant or insertion of C wires. If the implant does not fit, the distal end of the silicone prosthesis can be cut off to accommodate the fusion wire.

POSTOPERATIVE MANAGEMENT

Postoperatively the thumb is placed in a radial gutter splint for 10 days and then in a handbased thumb spica cast for 4 to 5 weeks. At that time,

dorsal apparatus off the underlying capsule as is necessary in MCP exposure of fingers in RA. Soft tissue balancing is unnecessary for the same reason. In the thumb MCP joint, the collateral ligaments can be recessed slightly, leaving their proximal attachments intact. A smaller portion of the metacarpal head can be removed, often measuring only 2 to 3 mm. Similarly, minimal bone can be removed from the base of the proximal phalanx. Then the largest prosthesis that fits is inserted, usually of a size 4, 5, or 6.

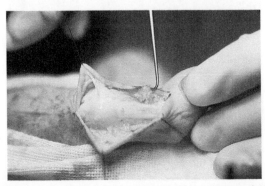

Fig. 5. Superficial dorsal exposure of the MCP and IP joints.

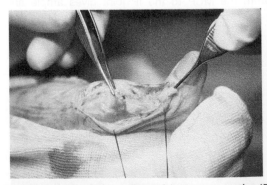

Fig. 7. Release of the collateral ligaments at the IP joint makes exposure easier.

the MCP joint no longer needs immobilization, but the presence or absence of an IP fusion determines the need for further immobilization by either cast or splint. Rehabilitation to increase MCP motion is desirable, but it is rare to achieve more than 20° to 30° of MCP motion. However, this range of motion is more than adequate to allow excellent function. At the IP level, usually the crossed pins and sometimes the intramedullary pin inconvenience patients enough that the pins have to be removed. Work on an entirely intramedullary device is proceeding.

EXPECTED RESULTS

Ferlic and colleagues[8] reported on the treatment of patients with destruction of both the MCP and IP joints. They fused the IP joint and used hinged metal prosthesis (the Flatt prosthesis) at the MCP joint. Although they reported favorable early assaults, long-term follow-up has shown unacceptable complications with a rigid metal hinge.

A Swanson-type silicone spacer has been used successfully for arthroplasty of the thumb MCP joint in RA. Figgie and colleagues[9] reported on a series of 59 implants in thumbs with less-severe IP arthritis. They found good relief of pain, reasonable maintenance of motion, and durable improvement in stability and pinch strength.

The authors' experience has reflected these findings. The results of these 2 procedures are excellent for pain relief, correction of deformity, and improvement of function. There are several advantages of MCP arthroplasty compared with MCP arthrodesis, one of which is preserving motion. It also eliminates concern about nonunion and many problems with painful hardware. Improved appearance after MCP arthroplasty is a major component of patient satisfaction.[10]

REFERENCES

1. Nalebuff EA. Diagnosis, classification and management of rheumatoid thumb deformities. Bull Hosp Joint Dis 1968;29(2):119–37.
2. Belt E, Kaarela K, Lehtinen J, et al. When does subluxation of the first carpometacarpal joint cause swan-neck deformity of the thumb in rheumatoid arthritis: a 20-year follow-up study. Clin Rheumatol 1998;17(2):135–8.
3. Zijlstra TR, Heijnsdijk-Rouwenhorst L, Rasker JJ. Silver ring splints improve dexterity in patients with rheumatoid arthritis. Arthritis Rheum 2004;51(6): 947–51.
4. Silva PG, Lombardi I Jr, Breitschwerdt C, et al. Functional thumb orthosis for type I and II boutonnière deformity on the dominant hand in patients with rheumatoid arthritis: a randomized controlled study. Clin Rehabil 2008;22(8):684–9.
5. Bliddal H, Terslev L, Qvistgaard E, et al. A randomized, controlled study of a single intra-articular injection of etanercept or glucocorticosteroids in patients with rheumatoid arthritis. Scand J Rheumatol 2006;35(5):341–5.
6. Terrono A, Millender L, Nalebuff E. Boutonnière rheumatoid thumb deformity. J Hand Surg Am 1990; 15(6):999–1003.
7. Nalebuff EA, Millender LH. Surgical treatment of the swan-neck deformity in rheumatoid arthritis. Orthop Clin North Am 1975;6(3):733–52.
8. Ferlic DC, Serot DI, Clayton ML. The use of the Flatt hinge prosthesis in the rheumatoid thumb. Hand 1978;10(1):94–8.
9. Figgie MP, Inglis AE, Sobel M, et al. Metacarpal-phalangeal joint arthroplasty of the rheumatoid thumb. J Hand Surg Am 1990;15(2):210–6.
10. Mandl LA, Galvin DH, Bosch JP, et al. Metacarpophalangeal arthroplasty in rheumatoid arthritis: what determines satisfaction with surgery? J Rheumatol 2002;29(12):2488–91.

The Rheumatoid Metacarpophalangeal Joint

Frank D. Burke, MBBS, FRCS

KEYWORDS

- Rheumatoid arthritis • Metacarpophalangeal joint
- Arthroplasty • Arthrodesis

The need for surgical intervention in rheumatoid hand deformities has been, to an extent, modified in recent years. This is in response to improved medical management involving the use of powerful new therapeutic agents. Progression of disease may be halted or slowed and the foreshortened fingers arising from premature epiphyseal closure in Still disease (juvenile idiopathic arthritis) is now a rarity. Nevertheless, conservative management will not control some cases and metacarpophalangeal (MP) joint reconstruction is still required for these patients.

THE CAUSES OF RHEUMATOID METACARPOPHALANGEAL DEFORMITIES

Twenty years ago, I treated a patient with rheumatoid arthritis with hand deformities. In her late teens, she sustained injuries riding a motorcycle. There was substantial bone loss at the right elbow; the wounds healed, leaving a flail right elbow and, somewhat unusually, no associated distal neurologic deficit. Five years later, she developed rheumatoid arthritis and was referred to me 5 years after that diagnosis had been confirmed. She presented with rheumatoid hand deformities. The flail right upper limb was worn in a silk scarf sling and its use was limited to feeding objects into the hand from the left hand. Use for the activities of daily living was minimal, with the left hand taking on almost all the functions of both upper limbs. There were severe rheumatoid deformities to the left upper limb in contrast to the right, which had no deformities. The patient offered a very obvious indication of the role of the activities of daily living in the development of rheumatoid hand deformities.

VOLAR SUBLUXATION OF THE PROXIMAL PHALANX BASE

Flatt and Ellison[1] described the force vectors arising when an object is held between the thumb and index fingertips (**Fig. 1**): 1 kg force applied to the object gives rise to 6 kg in the line of the long digital flexors with a 3-kg volar vector applied across the MP joint. This persistent force on use attenuates the incompetent rheumatoid soft tissue restraints to the MP joint, creating progressive volar subluxation to the base of the proximal phalanx (**Fig. 2**) with respect to the metacarpal head. Total dislocation may occur and the base of the proximal phalanx will then drift proximally, creating shortening to the digits and making reconstructive procedures more difficult (**Fig. 3**).

Ulnar Drift

Many distal rheumatoid hand deformities can be explained by more proximal joint malalignment. Synovitis of the wrist and attenuation of the ligaments may lead to the patient with rheumatoid arthritis maintaining the wrist in radial deviation. Radial tilt at the carpus creates a significant ulnar deviating force to the MP joints. This is evidenced by the effect of surgery to correct ulnar drift of the fingers in cases where a fusion of the wrist has been performed in the past and bone union has occurred in radial deviation of the carpus. The benefits of ulnar drift correction are likely to be short lived in these cases if the position of the wrist is left unchanged.

Pinch and chuck grip create ulnar deviating forces to the digits during activities of daily living.

The author has nothing to disclose.
Pulvertaft Hand Centre, Royal Derby Hospital, Uttoxeter Road 28 Midland Place, Derby DE22 3NE 5, UK
E-mail address: frank.burke@virgin.net

hand.theclinics.com

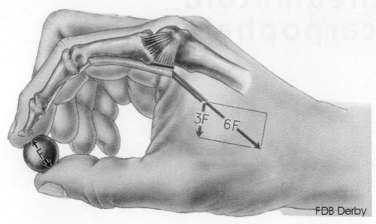

Fig. 1. The biomechanics of thumb index pinch. (*Reprinted from* Flatt AE. The care of the rheumatoid hand kinesiology. St Louis (MO): C V Mosby Company; 1974. p. 29; with permission.)

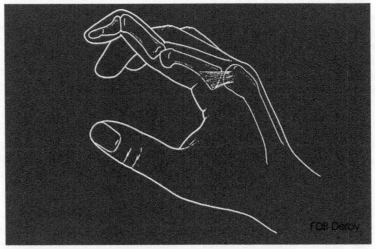

Fig. 2. Volar subluxation of the proximal phalanx. (*Reprinted from* Flatt AE. The care of the rheumatoid hand kinesiology. St Louis (MO): C V Mosby Company; 1974. p. 29; with permission.)

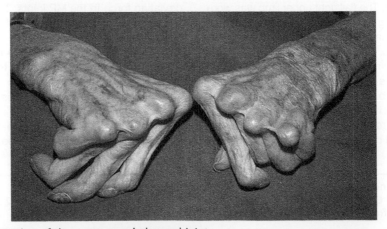

Fig. 3. Volar dislocation of the metacarpophalangeal joint.

In addition, there are mild ulnar vector forces to the index and long fingers as the flexor tendons traverse the palm from the carpal tunnel. Attenuation of the retinacular fibers maintaining the extensor tendons over the metacarpal head frequently lead to the extensor tendons migrating into the valleys to the ulnar side of the metacarpal head. This creates an additional ulnar vector, which will play a role in the development and severity of ulnar drift.

CARE PATHWAYS WHEN CONSIDERING SURGICAL OPTIONS

It is beyond the remit of this article to discuss the medical management of MP rheumatoid deformities. Two pathways need to be considered:

1. Direct referral to a surgeon from primary care.
2. Referral arising out of a combined clinic with rheumatologists.

The latter is the preferred management option, where rheumatologists, hand surgeons, and hand therapists meet in a combined clinic setting to provide consistent informed advice to the patient with rheumatoid arthritis and where the patient's often unique functional difficulties can be analyzed. Informed advice is not readily available for patients with rheumatoid arthritis. Alderman and colleagues[2] noted major differences in opinion between American hand surgeons and rheumatologists when a variety of upper limb rheumatoid surgery procedures were assessed for their efficacy. Surgeons, perhaps predictably, have greater confidence in the value of the procedures. In a similar study in the United Kingdom, as yet unpublished, a similar, but less polarized trend was noted. In the UK study, hand therapists were also asked their views on the efficacy of the index procedures. Their assessment usually lay between the views of surgeons and rheumatologists.

HAND THERAPY ASSESSMENT AND MANAGEMENT

The subject is beyond the immediate remit of this article and this issue of the journal, but it is an essential part of the optimized care pathway for a rheumatoid combined clinic. The patient benefits from functional assessment in workshop and kitchen, with application of aids and appliances appropriate to their needs to minimize functional difficulties and to maximize independence. Therapists also have a valuable role in advising on possible surgical options and can often usefully act as patient advocates when decisions are being made about choice of surgery. Their involvement can optimize the consenting process.

JOINT PROTECTION EXERCISES AND SPLINTS

Resting night splints to correct ulnar deviation of the MP joint can be applied. Their effectiveness at controlling deformity is uncertain and patient compliance may also be a difficulty. Dynamic splints can be worn during the day with slings under the proximal phalanges to draw the base of the proximal phalanx dorsally and the digits radially, thereby overcoming volar subluxation and ulnar deviation. Compliance with such regimes and the enthusiasm for their use are varied. The technique is widely used in northern European countries but less frequently used in the United Kingdom and North America.

MP Joint Synovectomy and Joint Realignment

The technique was used quite frequently 30 years ago but is used less frequently now, although this surgical option retains support in several countries in northern Europe. There is a strong tendency in North America and the United Kingdom to delay surgical intervention in these cases until joint replacement is considered to be necessary. Joint synovectomy involves exposing the joint through 3 possible incisions. A transverse incision can be used over the metacarpal heads; alternatively, 4 longitudinal incisions can be used directly over the metacarpal head or 2 longitudinal incisions each between a pair of metacarpal heads. The capsule is incised on the radial side and synovectomy performed, preserving the joint capsule. The extensor tendons are released from the valleys to the ulnar side of the metacarpal head and relocated onto the metacarpal head. The radial collateral ligament can be reefed or the radial portion of the volar plate sutured dorsally to overcome volar subluxation of the base of the proximal phalanx. The hand is rested on a volar slab with an ulnar gutter for a few days and then mobilized in a dynamic splint by day, maintaining correction of the ulnar drift and volar subluxation, for 8 to 10 weeks. A static night splint is worn for several months, seeking to maintain the correction.

MP JOINT ARTHROPLASTY FOR PATIENTS WITH RHEUMATOID ARTHRITIS
The History of Joint Arthroplasty

Colonel Brannon and Klein[3] designed a metal-hinged prosthesis for use at the MP and proximal interphalangeal (PIP) joint level. In 1959, they reported on a 14-patient series (all but 2 involving the PIP joint). All were young service personnel and most retained a satisfactory result with a moderate range of motion. I had the opportunity to see one of the implants removed in Louisville in 1976 (**Fig. 4**). The half-threaded rivet screw had fractured but the patient had maintained good function for 20 years. In 1961, Flatt[4] reported on a stainless steel implant for MP or PIP joint use (**Fig. 5**) and reviewed the results of 242 prostheses in 1972. MP joint range of motion was limited with a tendency to bone erosion. The implants were considered to offer stability with limited movement, and the use in 1976, when I worked in Iowa City, was restricted to the rheumatoid MP joint of the thumb.

In the years that followed the development of Flatt's implant, research into alternative designs split into 2 broad streams: the use of the Swanson silicone joint spacer, and the development of true implants constrained or unconstrained, seeking to emulate the now excellent results of total hip replacement. Many of the designs were under biomechanical evaluation in Iowa during my tenure (Gillespie and colleagues[5]). The sophisticated design of almost all these implants failed to deliver the intended benefit and the Steffee, the St George Buchholz, the Schultz, and the Strickland were withdrawn from use.

The Swanson joint replacement, considered by many to be a stop-gap implant until a "proper" joint was available, continued to offer benefits for patients with rheumatoid hand deformities and was recognized as an option that was safe and beneficial to patients, particularly if their requirements were low demand. More durable high-performance silicone was introduced to reduce

the risk of implant fracture and, in more recent years, alternative designs to the Swanson model have also gained acceptance (the Sutter, the Avanta, and the Neuflex). I continued to use the Swanson implant for patients with rheumatoid arthritis requiring MP joint arthroplasty.

A further generation of MP joint arthroplasties has been developed in recent years but assessment of benefits is clouded in most publications by the investigators offering relatively short-term reviews and tending to include PIP joint arthroplasties with those applied to the MP joint. The studies often also include rheumatoid and osteoarthritic cases. The longer-term benefit specifically to patients with rheumatoid arthritis at the MP joint remains uncertain. Kujula and colleagues[6] noted gratifying results but the study was limited to 7 implants in 2 patients reviewed at 10 months. Parker and colleagues[7] indicated short-term pain relief and a modest gain in motion, but with the risk of axial subsidence and erosions, particularly in patients with rheumatoid arthritis. Parker and colleagues[7] observed that nonconstrained pyrolytic carbon implants rely on stable soft tissue restraints around the joint. These usually are available in cases involving osteoarthritis but are commonly deficient in cases presenting with rheumatoid arthritis. Cook and colleagues[8] offered a large pyrocarbon implant series of cases (26) reviewed at an average of 11.5 years. Twelve percent of a larger series had required revision. Eighty percent of cases suffered from rheumatoid arthritis. The survival rate was 82% at 5 years and 81% at 10 years. Of the 71 implants available for review, 34 were noted to have exhibited mild to

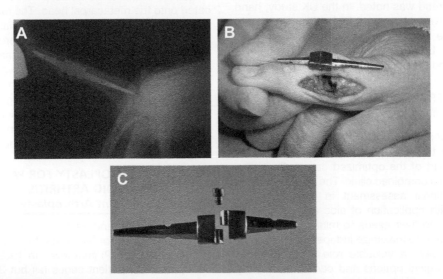

Fig. 4. (A–C). Brannon prosthesis.

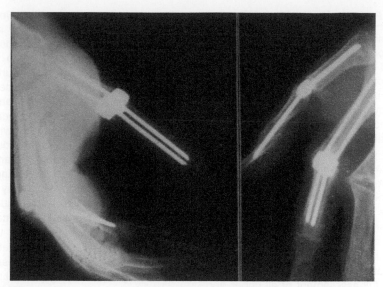

Fig. 5. Flatt prothesis.

moderate subsidence. Recurrent volar subluxation did not seem to be a significant problem with these patients but ulnar deviation was noted to recur to previous levels (average 20° preoperatively and 19° at review). Surgery reduced the extensor lag and this benefit was noted to be retained to long-term review. The postoperative range of motion increased modestly with further additional gains at long-term review.

The long-term outcome for Swanson joint replacements has been documented reasonably well by Chung and colleagues[9] in a systematic review and by Goldfarb and Stern[10] and Trail and colleagues.[11] The procedure offers good pain relief and a modest increase in range of motion, which tends to decrease over time. The arc of motion shifts to a position of greater extension. Implant fractures did not necessarily create a need for revision and rates of revision surgery were low.

A limited number of articles have investigated the benefits of alternative silicone implants. Parkkila and colleagues[12] did not find any appreciable difference between Sutter implants and the Swanson joint replacement. Delaney and colleagues[13] compared the Neuflex implant against the Swanson and found a greater range of motion with the Neuflex, but the study was small and limited to 2-year review. Moller and colleagues[14] compared the Avanta silicone implant with the Swanson. A modest increase in range at 2-year review occurred when the Avanta had been used, but the implant was associated with a higher fracture rate.

Currently the guest editor of this edition of *Hand Clinics* has been leading a multicenter study reviewing the middle-term outcome (7 years) of Swanson MP joint arthroplasty contrasting their outcome with a similar group of patients who elected at the outset to continue nonoperative care by rheumatologists. Enrollment is complete but the study has 2 more years to run. Preliminary results reveal those seeking surgery were generally more disabled by the rheumatoid process and the operative intervention lifted their function (1 year after surgery) to the functional level of those who had elected to enter the nonoperative limb of the study. Grip and pinch were not improved by surgery. The medical wing of the study maintained functional status at the first-year review with no observable deterioration in function. Swanson arthroplasty outcome was not undermined by more severe ulnar drift preoperatively; they gained a greater correction. One study center has investigated the relationship between early postoperative complications and concomitant chemotherapy. Only one type of drug was stopped before the surgery (Etanercept, discontinued 2–3 weeks preoperatively). All other medications (nonsteroidal anti-inflammatories biologics, cytotoxics, noncytotoxics, and steroids) were continued over the operative period. There were no serious problems to the 140 wounds studied. Four minor problems occurred (slightly delayed wound healing, suture granuloma, a rheumatoid flare, and a possible superficial wound infection) and all settled satisfactorily.

Assessment of Patients for Surgery

The combined clinic model with rheumatologists and hand therapists is preferred. The principles Souter[15] offered in 1979 are still relevant. The mere existence of deformity is not necessarily an indication for surgery. Surgeon and therapist need to look beyond the deformity and assess the disability and whether surgical options will likely improve matters. Decisions should be paced with a patient empowered by knowledge of surgery, rehabilitation, and likely outcome. A separate assessment by therapists in a workshop/kitchen environment is valuable.

Particular care has to be taken to assess the viability of the skin to the dorsum of the hand. Splinter hemorrhages to the nail beds may question the skin's ability to heal with compromised rehabilitation postoperatively or implant exposure and infection. A full assessment of all upper and lower limbs is required to ensure the anticipated benefit at MP joint level will not be undermined by other problems. Patients with rheumatoid arthritis are often candidates for several surgical options at any given time. These options need to be prioritized to the patients' needs. Patients need to "gear-up" to elective surgery and most patients with rheumatoid arthritis are reluctant to sign up for more than one operative procedure in a year.

Operative Technique

Patients are preclerked and attend on the day of surgery. Anesthesia is usually by brachial block or general anesthesia if preferred. The limb is prepped and draped with an upper arm tourniquet in place. Care is taken to ensure the preparation agent does not seep under the tourniquet (I prefer exsanguination using a sterile crepe bandage that will be used at the end of the procedure as part of the dressing). The small amount of blood that is left in the vessels facilitates identification. I prefer 4 longitudinal incisions over the MP joints with a similar incision to the retinacular fibers, which are attenuated on top of the joint. The retinacular fibers should then be dissected off the joint capsule. The capsule is then incised and mobilized sufficiently for a fulsome view of the metacarpal head and neck. Synovectomy is performed; the extent of head and neck resection is variable. Preoperative radiographs will help give some information as to the degree of proximal phalanx base subluxation and proximal migration under the metacarpal head. Minor migration may permit resection of the metacarpal head, preserving the collateral ligament origins, but this will not be possible with more severe deformity. Resect the head and complete the synovectomy if required. Drill a hole in the proximal phalanx base to allow the entry of a Swanson reamer to square off the cortical defect to the articular surface to accommodate the base of the stem. The medulla of the proximal phalanx can then be reamed.

I prefer to compact the metacarpal medullary bone and only ream the cavity when the bone is very narrow (most commonly found in the ring metacarpal). The largest implant is preferred based on what will fit in the metacarpal; it would be unusual to find sizing limited by the dimensions of the proximal phalanx. Trial reductions are helpful to check that enough metacarpal head has been excised. Undue tightness will limit flexion postoperatively; be aware that silicone trial implants shrink slightly as a result of repetitive autoclaving and a very tight trial fit probably means the implant chosen will be slightly too big. The implant is inserted into the metacarpal and then fed into the proximal phalanx base with nontoothed forceps with the joint held in flexion. I do not use grommets (Trail and colleagues[11] did not find they improved outcome). If the implant is seated satisfactorily, I may reef the radial collateral ligament with a nonabsorbable suture. I am not in the habit of mobilizing part of the volar plate dorsally to overcome volar subluxation. The extensor tendon is then released, on its ulnar border, and relocated over the implant and the retinacular fibers reefed to maintain the position. The skin is closed without drains. I prefer to operate on the fingers in twos, first the index and middle fingers with skin closure to both before starting on the ring and little fingers. Paraffin gauze and dressings are applied and the hand rested on a volar slab with an ulnar gutter to avoid ulnar deviation. The hand is then elevated with firm pressure over the wound and the tourniquet released and removed immediately, to avoid the risk of venous congestion during the phase of reactive hyperemia. Elevation with a near straight elbow and firm pressure to the operative area is continued for 3 to 4 minutes, when the reactive hyperemia is at its maximum. There were no hematomas in the 140 wounds treated by this method in our recent case series nor do I recall hematoma problems in the past. The patient is discharged that evening with dressing changes at 3 to 5 days and the creation of a static night splint to maintain MP joint extension and the avoidance of ulnar deviation. An extensor outrigger is applied for daytime use, holding the MP joints in extension with a radial force applied to mold the scar tissue in the early weeks from surgery. The dynamic splint is used for 6 to 8 weeks, depending on

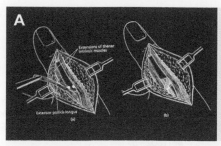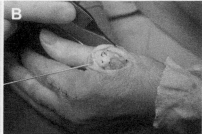

Fig. 6. (*A, B*) Extensor pollicis longus to extensor pollicis brevis transfer.

progress and the static splint 10 to 12 weeks or longer if patients prefer.

THE MP JOINT OF THE THUMB

Boutonniere and swan neck deformities have the effect of shortening the effective length of the thumb, thereby reducing precision skills. Stability takes precedence over mobility at the MP joint and arthrodesis presents a popular option, offering predictable lasting benefit. A longitudinal dorsal incision over the MP joint affords a good view of the joint; the incision is deepened to the joint and the sides of the proximal phalanx base and metacarpal head are exposed. A limited excision of the head is performed with the plane of the excision in 10° of flexion with respect to the long axis of the first metacarpal. A minimum of bone is then excised from the proximal phalanx base, cut perpendicular to the long axis of the bone. If bone stock is judged to be reasonable, fixation with an oblique Kirschner (K)-wire and a cerclage wire is adequate and involves minimal hardware, which does not lie too close to the skin. The disparity in width between metacarpal head and proximal phalanx base allow for the twisted portion of the cerclage wire to lie in an unobtrusive area down the side of the fusion site. The K-wire is passed distally until it bites into the proximal phalanx cortex and the proximal end is then bent over, cut short, and rotated to lie as flat as possible. The internal fixation can then be ignored with no need for removal after bone union. Patients with rheumatoid arthritis suffer so many difficulties in life that any surgical technique that offers them simple postoperative care is to be recommended. If bone stock is considered to be poor, tension band wiring offers improved stability with minimal additional hardware.

Extensor Pollicis Longus to Extensor Pollicis Brevis Transfer

A minority of patients present for assessment with a boutonniere deformity to the MP joint of the thumb, where radiographs reveal a fairly satisfactory joint surface and the joint is stable. Thumb length can be regained and joint mobility preserved with an underused surgical option (**Fig. 6**). The extensor pollicis longus is mobilized, leaving the soft tissues on its immediate margins in longitudinal continuity. It is released from the distal phalanx. A mallet deformity will not occur if the soft tissues on the immediate margins of the tendon are preserved. A drill hole is then made near the base of the proximal phalanx and the tendon drawn through and sutured under tension to itself. Active extension of the MP joint is regained with improved thumb length and dexterity. The new tendon insertion is usually robust, which allows early movement postoperatively.

SUMMARY

Swanson MP joint arthroplasty remains a beneficial operative intervention in carefully selected cases. The combined clinic with rheumatologists is the preferred environment in which these cases should be considered. Hand therapists offer valuable additional benefits in terms of optimized care (advice on splints and appliances) and patient advocacy during the consenting process. The role of the latest generation of pyrocarbon implants applied to the rheumatoid MP joint remains uncertain. The vulnerability of the patient with rheumatoid arthritis to attenuation of ligaments may undermine any lasting benefit with pyrocarbon implants through joint subluxation, recurrent ulnar drift, and bone erosion around the implant stem.

REFERENCES

1. Flatt AE, Ellison MR. Restoration of rheumatoid finger function III: a follow-up note after 14 years of experience with a metallic hinge prosthesis. J Bone Joint Surg Am 1972;54:1317–22.
2. Alderman AK, Chung KC, Kim HM, et al. Effectiveness of rheumatoid hand surgery: contrasting

perceptions of hand surgeons and rheumatologists. J Hand Surg Am 2003;28:3–11.

3. Brannon EW, Klein G. Experiences with a finger joint prosthesis. J Bone Joint Surg Am 1959;41:87–102.

4. Flatt AE. Restoration of rheumatoid finger joint function: interim report on trial of prosthetic replacement. J Bone Joint Surg Am 1961;42:753–74.

5. Gillespie TE, Flatt AE, Youm Y, et al. Biomechanical evaluation of metacarpophalangeal joint prosthesis designs. J Hand Surg Am 1979;4:508–21.

6. Kujala S, Bongiorno V, Leppilahti J, et al. Pyrolytic carbon MCP arthroplasty: a report of seven prostheses implanted into two patients. J Orthop Traumatol 2006;7(1):12–5.

7. Parker WL, Rizzo M, Moran SL, et al. Preliminary results of non constrained pyrolytic carbon arthroplasty for metacarpophalangeal joint arthritis. J Hand Surg Am 2007;32:1496–505.

8. Cook SD, Beckenbaugh RD, Redondo J, et al. Long-term follow-up of pyrolyctic carbon metacarpophalangeal implants. J Bone Joint Surg Am 1999;81:635–48.

9. Chung KC, Kowalski CP, Kim HM, et al. Patient outcomes following Swanson silastic metacarpophalangeal joint arthroplasty in the rheumatoid hand: a systematic overview. J Rheumatol 2000;27(6):1395–402.

10. Goldfarb CA, Stern PJ. Metacarpophalangeal joint arthroplasty in rheumatoid arthritis. J Bone Joint Surg Am 2003;85:1869–78.

11. Trail IA, Martin JA, Nuttall D, et al. Seventeen years survivorship analysis of silastic metacarpophalangeal joint replacement. J Bone Joint Surg Br 2004;86:1002–6.

12. Parkkila T, Belt EA, Hakaka M, et al. Comparison of Swanson and Sutter metacarpophalangeal joint arthroplasties in patients with rheumatoid arthritis: a prospective and randomised trial. J Hand Surg Am 2005;30:1276–81.

13. Delaney R, Trail IA, Nuttall D. A comparative study of outcome between the neuflex and Swanson metacarpophalangeal joint replacements. J Hand Surg Br 2005;30:3–7.

14. Moller K, Sollerman C, Geijer M, et al. Avanta versus Swanson silicon implants in the MCP joint. Randomised comparison of 30 patients followed for 2 years. J Hand Surg Br 2005;30:8–13.

15. Souter WE. Planning treatment of the rheumatoid hand. Hand 1979;11:3–16.

Reconstruction of Digital Deformities in Rheumatoid Arthritis

Sandeep J. Sebastin, MCh[a], Kevin C. Chung, MD, MS[b,*]

KEYWORDS

- Rheumatoid arthritis • Digital deformities
- Swan neck deformity • Boutonnière deformity
- Flexor tenosynovitis

Rheumatoid arthritis (RA) is a disease of the synovial membrane, and the resultant inflammatory synovitis is directly or indirectly responsible for the deformities seen in the digits.[1] An untreated rheumatoid digital deformity transforms from a passively correctable flexible deformity to a deformity with limited motion and finally a fixed deformity. Although the initial inciting factor is synovitis, the progression of the digital deformity results from a combination of synovitis, adhesions, shortening and/or rupture of the ligaments, intrinsic muscles, and extrinsic tendons, leading to poor joint position and joint ankylosis. When evaluating digital deformities for surgical treatment, the surgeon needs to classify them into flexible or fixed deformities. Although many options are available for the treatment of flexible deformities, these options become progressively limited with increasing joint stiffness, and joint fusion is the only reliable option for a fixed interphalangeal joint deformity in RA. For a deformed digit with limited motion, the aim is to recover flexibility first.

The 2 classic digital deformities seen in RA are swan neck deformity (SND) and boutonnière deformity (BND) (**Fig. 1**).[2] The incidence of uncorrectable SND and BND is estimated to be between 8% and 16% during the first 2 years after the onset of systemic disease, and the prevalence of finger deformities in patients with established RA is approximately 14% for SND and 36% for BND.[3] Although both conditions occur at the proximal interphalangeal joint (PIPJ), an SND can result from synovitis at the wrist, metacarpophalangeal joint (MCPJ), PIPJ, or the distal interphalangeal joint (DIPJ), whereas a BND always results from PIPJ synovitis. It is not uncommon for the same hand to develop both deformities simultaneously (see **Fig. 1**A).[4] A patient with an SND is unable to make a full fist because of the hyperextended posture of the PIPJ, whereas a patient with a BND is able to make a fist but is unhappy with the flexed posture of the PIPJ when the digit is extended (see **Fig. 1**B). An SND, therefore, causes a functional problem, whereas a BND is more of an aesthetic concern. The surgical treatment of an SND places the digit in a functional posture, whereas the treatment of BND risks changing the flexed posture of the PIPJ into a functionally limiting extended posture.

Although most attention in rheumatoid digits is directed toward the evaluation of SNDs and BNDs, one must not forget to examine the digit for the presence of other rheumatoid changes. The concomitant conditions can include flexor tenosynovitis that can lead to trigger digits and rupture of the flexor tendons and synovitis of the interphalangeal joints. The treatment of these

Supported in part by a Midcareer Investigator Award in Patient-Oriented Research (K24 AR053120) from the National Institute of Arthritis and Musculoskeletal and Skin Diseases (to Dr Kevin C. Chung).

[a] Department of Hand and Reconstructive Microsurgery, National University Health System, 1E Kent Ridge Road, NUHS Tower Block, Level 11, Singapore 119228
[b] Section of Plastic Surgery, Department of Surgery, University of Michigan Medical School, 2130 Taubman Center, SPC 5340, 1500 East Medical Center Drive, Ann Arbor, MI 48109-5340, USA
* Corresponding author.
E-mail address: kecchung@umich.edu

Hand Clin 27 (2011) 87–104
doi:10.1016/j.hcl.2010.10.006
0749-0712/11/$ — see front matter © 2011 Elsevier Inc. All rights reserved.

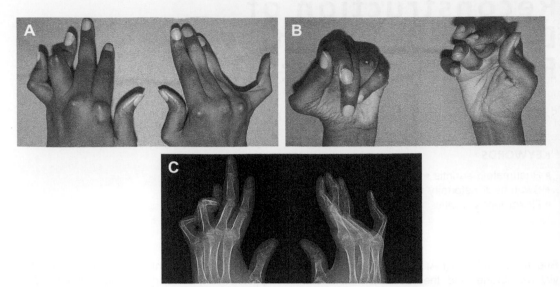

Fig. 1. A 40-year-old patient with bilateral rheumatoid hand deformities. (*A*) Boutonnière deformities of left small, left ring, and right small fingers with simultaneous swan neck deformities of left long, right long, and right ring fingers. (*B*) Note inability to make a fist on the right hand (predominantly swan neck deformity) compared with the left hand (predominantly boutonnière deformity). (*C*) Radiograph.

conditions when detected early is rewarding. The correction of digital deformities is last in the priority of surgical procedures for the rheumatoid hand and wrist. The surgical treatment of the rheumatoid wrist, MCPJ, and thumb deformities takes priority because the results are good and these procedures contribute significantly to improving the quality of life. The results of surgery in rheumatoid SND and BND are unpredictable, and the patient may regain adequate function once the proximal deformities have been addressed or adapt quite well to the disease, despite obvious digital deformities. Surgery for digital deformities can predictably improve function only in a few patients with RA, and the surgeon must consider the outcome carefully before offering surgical correction.

ANATOMY AND KINEMATICS

An appreciation of the anatomy and kinematics of the extensor apparatus is essential for understanding the pathogenesis and treatment of the rheumatoid digital deformities.[5–7] The extensor apparatus is composed of a musculotendinous system and a ligamentous system. The musculotendinous system comprises the radial nerve–innervated extrinsic extensors (extensor digitorum communis, extensor indicis proprius, and extensor digiti minimi quinti) and the intrinsic muscles (palmar interossei [PI], dorsal interossei [DI], and lumbrical muscles) supplied by the ulnar and median nerves. The ligamentous system

comprises of 4 ligaments, namely the sagittal band, triangular ligament, transverse retinacular ligament (TRL), and oblique retinacular ligament (ORL). These ligaments maintain equilibrium between the intrinsic and extrinsic musculotendinous systems.

Musculotendinous System

Extensor tendon

As the extrinsic extensor tendon passes over the MCPJ, it becomes flattened and bandlike. At the junction of the proximal and middle third of the proximal phalanx, it divides into 3 slips: a central slip and 2 lateral slips. The central slip continues in the midline, and at the level of the neck of the proximal phalanx, it receives the medial band of the intrinsic tendon on both sides. It then continues as the central band, which inserts into the base of the dorsal aspect of the middle phalanx. Each lateral slip merges with the respective lateral bands of the intrinsic tendon to form a conjoint lateral band. The conjoint lateral bands on both sides join with each other on the dorsum of the finger at the level of the middle and distal third of the middle phalanx, forming the terminal tendon, which inserts onto the dorsal aspect of the base of the distal phalanx. The extensor tendon is considered to have 2 more insertions in addition to the 2 described earlier. The first is onto the lateral aspect of the volar plate of the MCPJ via the sagittal band. The second is by an inconstant slip from the deep surface of the tendon to the base of the dorsal aspect of the proximal phalanx (**Figs. 2** and **3**).[7]

Interossei

There are 3 palmar and 4 dorsal interosseous muscles. The interossei originate between the metacarpal shafts and insert into the base of the proximal phalanx and the lateral band. The interosseous tendon passes volar to the axis of the MCPJ but remains dorsal to the deep transverse metacarpal ligament, contributes fibers to the sagittal band, and forms the intrinsic tendon (see **Fig. 3**). On the ulnar side of the digit, the intrinsic tendon is formed by the tendons of the PI and DI, whereas on the radial side, it is formed by the interossei (palmar and dorsal) and the lumbrical tendon (see **Fig. 2**). At the junction of the proximal and middle third of the proximal phalanx, each intrinsic tendon divides into the medial and lateral bands. The medial band joins with the central slip of the extensor tendon to form the central band, and the lateral band joins with the lateral slips of the extensor tendon to form the conjoint lateral band (see **Figs. 2** and **3**).

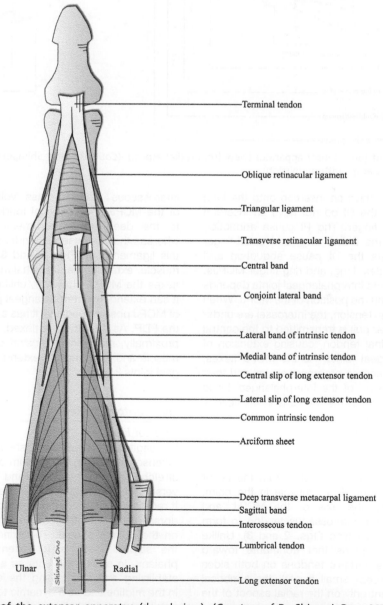

Terminal tendon

Oblique retinacular ligament

Triangular ligament

Transverse retinacular ligament

Central band

Conjoint lateral band

Lateral band of intrinsic tendon

Medial band of intrinsic tendon

Central slip of long extensor tendon

Lateral slip of long extensor tendon

Common intrinsic tendon

Arciform sheet

Deep transverse metacarpal ligament

Sagittal band

Interosseous tendon

Lumbrical tendon

Long extensor tendon

Ulnar   Radial

Shimpei Ono

Fig. 2. Anatomy of the extensor apparatus (dorsal view). (*Courtesy of* Dr Shimpei Ono, MD, Tokyo, Japan, s-ono@nms.ac.jp; with permission).

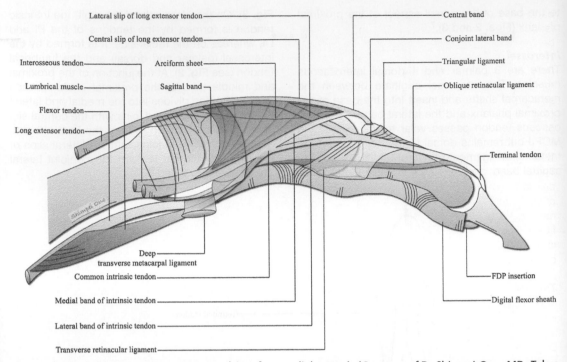

Fig. 3. Anatomy of the extensor apparatus (view from radial aspect). (*Courtesy of* Dr Shimpei Ono, MD, Tokyo, Japan, s-ono@nms.ac.jp; with permission).

The PI do not have an insertion onto the long finger, whereas the DI do not have an insertion onto the small finger. The PI cause adduction and flexion at the index, ring, and small-finger MCPJs, whereas the DI cause abduction and flexion of the index, long, and ring-finger MCPJs. Their action on the interphalangeal joints depends to some extent on the position of the MCPJ. When the MCPJ is in extension, the interossei are under tension, and their pull is transmitted to the central band and terminal tendon, causing extension of the interphalangeal joints. As the MCPJ flexes, the interossei become progressively lax and their action of extension of the interphalangeal joints decreases, and when the MCPJ is in full flexion, they no longer contribute to the extension of the interphalangeal joints.[7,8]

Lumbrical muscle

The lumbrical muscle originates from the flexor digitorum profundus (FDP) muscle in the palm, passes volar to the axis of the MCPJ, and combines with the interosseous tendon to form the intrinsic tendon (see **Figs. 2** and **3**). Unlike the interossei tendons that contribute toward formation of the intrinsic tendons on both sides of the digit (except small finger), the lumbrical tendon is present only on the radial aspect of the digit and contributes to formation of only the radial intrinsic tendon. Although both the lumbrical and

interosseous tendons pass volar to the axis of the MCPJ, the lumbrical tendon passes volar to the deep transverse metacarpal ligament, whereas the interosseous tendons pass dorsal to this ligament (see **Figs. 2** and **3**). The lumbrical muscle extends the interphalangeal joints and flexes the MCPJ. However, unlike the interossei, it can extend the interphalangeal joint irrespective of MCPJ position because it has a mobile origin on the FDP. As the MCPJ is flexed, the FDP moves proximally, maintaining tension on the lumbrical muscle and allowing it to extend the interphalangeal joints.[6]

Ligamentous System

Sagittal band

The sagittal band is a fibrous sheet that invests the extensor tendon on the dorsum of the MCPJ and stretches to the volar plate and the deep transverse metacarpal ligament on the palmar aspect. It receives fibers from the extensor tendon on the dorsal aspect and from the interosseous tendons on the palmar aspect. The principal function of the sagittal band is to extend the proximal phalanx. In addition, it acts as a static tether by stabilizing and maintaining the extensor tendon in the midline and as a dynamic tether by allowing proximal and distal gliding of the extensor tendons during finger flexion and extension. The sagittal band continues distally as a thin aponeurotic sheet (arciform sheet). This triangular sheet extends between the extensor tendon and the intrinsic tendon and is composed of a layered crisscross fiber pattern, which changes its geometric arrangement as the finger flexes and extends. This arrangement allows the intrinsic tendons to be displaced volarly in flexion and to return to the dorsum of the finger in extension (see **Figs. 2** and **3**).[9]

Triangular ligament

The triangular ligament is situated dorsally over the proximal half of the middle phalanx. It is composed of transverse fibers that extend between the medial sides of the conjoint lateral bands. The fibers maintain the dorsal position of the conjoint lateral bands and limit palmar and lateral shift during flexion of the PIPJ (see **Fig. 2**).

TRL

The TRL is situated on the lateral aspect of the proximal half of the middle phalanx. It consists of transverse fibers that extend from the lateral side of the conjoint lateral band to the volar plate of the PIPJ and the fibrous flexor sheath. These transverse fibers continue onto the dorsum, merging with the fibers of the triangular ligament. The TRL is superficial to the ORL and the collateral ligaments of the PIPJ. The main function of the TRL is to prevent dorsomedial shift of the conjoint lateral band when the finger is extended (see **Fig. 3**).

ORL

The ORL is situated on the lateral aspect of the digit and has an oblique volar-to-dorsal course. It begins on the lateral aspect of the proximal

phalanx and the fibrous flexor sheath at the level of the neck of the proximal phalanx and courses distally and dorsally. It passes volar to the axis of the PIPJ, superficial to the collateral ligament, deep to the TRL, and along the side of the middle phalanx and inserts into the conjoint lateral band at the level of the neck of the middle phalanx. It is consistently palmar to the PIPJ and dorsal to the DIPJ axis of rotation (see **Fig. 3**). The ORL is said to coordinate movement of the interphalangeal joints and act as a dynamic tenodesis to aid the conjoint lateral band in extension of the DIPJ.[10] Extension of the PIPJ places the ORL under tension and prevents easy active or passive flexion of the DIPJ.[11]

PATHOLOGY AND TREATMENT
SND

SND is characterized by hyperextension of the PIPJ, with reciprocal flexion of the MCPJ and DIPJ (**Fig. 4**).[12]

Pathogenesis

An SND can occur as a result of abnormalities at the wrist, MCPJ, PIPJ, or DIPJ. The key to the treatment of a flexible SND is to determine the joint that is primarily responsible for the development of the SND. It is therefore essential to understand how synovitis at each of these joints can lead to the development of an SND (**Fig. 5**).

Primary PIPJ pathology

The synovial lining of the PIPJ, especially the synovium within the palmar synovial pouch, becomes inflamed and hyperplastic to form a pannus, which distends the joint and stretches the dorsal surface

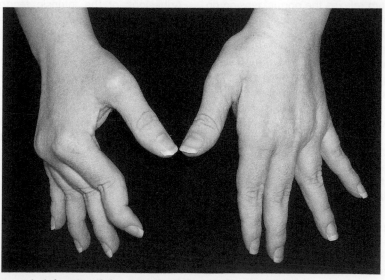

Fig. 4. Classic swan neck deformity of the right hand in a 42-year-old patient.

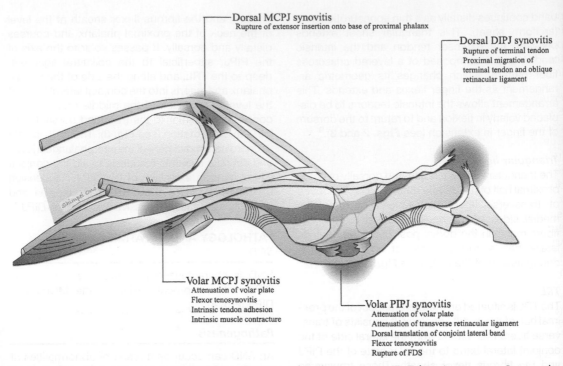

Dorsal MCPJ synovitis
Rupture of extensor insertion onto base of proximal phalanx

Dorsal DIPJ synovitis
Rupture of terminal tendon
Proximal migration of
terminal tendon and oblique
retinacular ligament

Volar MCPJ synovitis
Attenuation of volar plate
Flexor tenosynovitis
Intrinsic tendon adhesion
Intrinsic muscle contracture

Volar PIPJ synovitis
Attenuation of volar plate
Attenuation of transverse retinacular ligament
Dorsal translation of conjoint lateral band
Flexor tenosynovitis
Rupture of FDS

Fig. 5. Pathogenesis of a swan neck deformity. (*Courtesy of* Dr Shimpei Ono, MD, Tokyo, Japan, s-ono@nms.ac.jp; with permission).

of the volar plate, the check rein ligaments, and along the dorsal surface of the FDS tendon. Later, the FDP may also become involved, and the tendon sheath filled with hyperplastic tissue and free fluid. This synovitis leads to stretching, weakening, and eventually destruction of the volar plate and collateral ligaments and the insertion of the FDS, resulting in the loss of palmar restraint at the PIPJ. This loss allows the normal extensor forces to cause abnormal hyperextension of the PIPJ, which in turn relaxes the normal tension on the conjoint lateral bands, leading to dorsal migration.[13,14] A relaxed conjoint lateral band loses the ability to extend the DIPJ. In addition, the hyperextension of the PIPJ stretches the FDP, increasing its flexor action of the DIPJ, and causes the loss of the mechanical advantage of the ORL in extending the DIPJ. This loss of tension of the conjoint lateral band and ORL and increased tension of the FDP results in a DIPJ flexion deformity.[12] Over time, adhesions develop between the central slip and the dorsally translated conjoint lateral bands, converting the flexible deformity to a fixed deformity.

Primary MCPJ pathology

Synovitis of the MCPJ can lead to weakening of the insertion of the long extensors on the dorsal base of the proximal phalanx. This weakening transmits the extensor force to the base of the middle phalanx, resulting in hyperextension of the PIPJ. On the volar side, the synovitis causes attenuation of the volar plate, resulting in volar subluxation of the MCPJ. Over time, volar subluxation results in shortening of the intrinsic muscles, leading to PIPJ hyperextension and ultimately SND. This condition is compounded by synovitis in the flexor tendon sheath, which restricts flexor tendon excursion, concentrating the flexor force on the proximal phalanx, resulting in MCPJ flexion. Adhesions of the intrinsic tendons around the MCPJ from rheumatoid synovitis can also cause intrinsic contracture. A few investigators have proposed spasm of the intrinsic muscles to be the result of irritation from MCPJ synovitis, whereas others have suggested that the afferent pain stimuli from the inflamed MCPJ capsule triggers a protective pain reflex, which produces spasm in the intrinsic muscle supplied by the same spinal cord segment.[15] Secondary fibrosis in the persistently contracting muscle leads to contracture.

Primary DIPJ pathology

DIPJ synovitis can cause weakening and rupture of the terminal extensor tendon insertion, leading to the development of a mallet deformity. The proximal migration of the terminal extensor insertion causes the lateral bands to become lax. All the power of the common extrinsic extensor is now directed toward the central slip that inserts into the middle phalanx. Over time, the volar supporting structures of the PIPJ are weakened, and the PIPJ is forced into hyperextension, resulting in an SND.

Primary wrist pathology

Synovitis at the wrist joint can lead to carpal collapse, carpal supination, and ulnar translation. Carpal collapse leads to a relative lengthening (relaxation) of the long flexor and extensor tendons. The interosseous muscle can then overpower the action of the extrinsic muscles and lead to MCPJ flexion and PIPJ extension, which is aided by carpal supination and ulnar translation that lead to a flexion deformity at the wrist and the MCPJ. This deformity results in a posture of MCPJ flexion, which, over a prolonged period, causes a physiologic shortening of the intrinsic muscles.

Management

Although the pathogenesis seems quite complicated, the evaluation of an SND is simple and logical. The first step is to determine the passive range of motion at the PIPJ, which is used to classify the deformity in 1 of 3 types.

Full passive range of PIPJ motion

In patients with a normal range of passive PIPJ motion, the next step is to evaluate the MCPJ. The MCPJ is examined to determine the condition of the articular surfaces and the presence of intrinsic muscle shortening. Passive testing of joint stability helps in assessing attenuation or complete rupture of ligaments, and a grinding test may be done to determine the degree of joint cartilage damage. The degree of damage is better confirmed on a radiograph. The tightness of the intrinsic muscle is assessed using the Finochietto-Bunnell test.[16] This test examines the effect of MCPJ position on PIPJ flexion. Under normal circumstances, PIPJ flexion can be accomplished with the MCPJ fully extended. If the intrinsic muscles are shortened, PIPJ flexion is limited, as MCPJ extension increases. The test result is considered positive when there is less flexion of the PIPJ when the MCPJ is held extended than when the MCPJ is flexed (**Fig. 6**). One can test for shortening of the ulnar and radial intrinsic muscles by performing the test with the MCPJ alternately radially and ulnarly deviated. In cases with an associated ulnar drift deformity, the ulnar intrinsic muscles are shorter than the radial intrinsic muscles. However, the

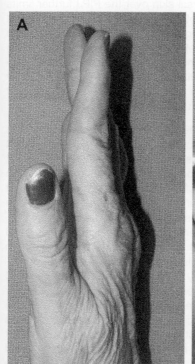
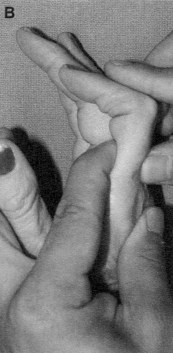
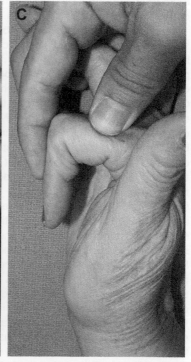

Fig. 6. Finochietto-Bunnell test for assessing intrinsic tightness. (*A*) A 67-year-old patient with a flexible swan neck deformity of the right index finger. (*B*) PIPJ flexion is restricted when the MCPJ is hyperextended. (*C*) Improved range of PIPJ flexion when the MCPJ is flexed.

radial intrinsic muscles are weaker and atrophic from lack of use.[17] In cases with long-standing intrinsic muscle shortening, extension of the MCPJ is not possible because of the secondary shortening of the capsular structures of the MCPJ, tightness of the palmar skin, and flexor tendon adhesions.

The DIPJ is evaluated next to determine the condition of the articular surfaces and if the insertion of the terminal tendon into the base of the dorsum of the distal phalanx is preserved. Stiffness at the DIPJ with grating on motion suggests articular damage, which can be confirmed by radiography. The integrity of the terminal tendon can be determined by asking the patient to actively extend the DIPJ, with the examiner correcting the PIPJ hyperextension.

Treatment The treatment of the MCPJ should take precedence in patients with an abnormal MCPJ. An intrinsic release for intrinsic contracture and/or MCPJ implant arthroplasty for MCPJ articular damage or volar subluxation should be done. If the articular surface of the MCPJ is preserved and there is no volar subluxation, but an ulnar drift deformity exists, the released radial intrinsic tendon can be used for a crossed intrinsic tendon transfer to correct the ulnar drift deformity of the adjacent long, ring, and small fingers. The treatment of an abnormal DIPJ (loss of terminal tendon or articular damage) is DIPJ fusion.

The surgical treatment of a flexible hyperextension deformity at the PIPJ aims to create a palmar restraint that allows flexion and extension but prevents hyperextension. A tenodesis is most often used for this purpose, which can be done using either the FDS (superficialis tenodesis)[18–20] or the conjoint lateral band.[10,21,22] Many variations of both have been described, and the choice between them is mostly a matter of personal preference. The most important aspect of tenodesis is to fix the tendon to the bone instead of to the soft tissue (eg, collateral ligament, pulley, flexor sheath), because a soft tissue attachment invariably attenuates over time. The authors prefer the superficialis tenodesis because the procedure is simple, provides a sturdier checkrein against PIPJ hyperextension, and can be done in the palm, thus avoiding dissection in zone 2.[23] The superficialis tenodesis does not address the mallet deformity in subjects with an intact terminal tendon insertion. The conjoint lateral band tenodesis corrects the PIPJ hyperextension and DIPJ flexion simultaneously. However, the quality of the conjoint lateral band can vary from patient to patient, and dissecting it in a rheumatoid digit can be challenging.

Technique of FDS tenodesis A zigzag incision is made on the volar aspect of the MCPJ. The triangular skin flap is raised, and both neurovascular bundles are identified and protected. The A1 pulley is identified, and the flexor sheath opened proximal to it. The FDS tendon is identified, and the radial slip of the FDS is divided 1 cm proximal to the A1 pulley and separated from the ulnar slip. A small bone anchor is inserted into the radial lateral aspect of the shaft of the metacarpal proximal to the neck. The divided slip of the FDS is sutured to the bone anchor in enough tension to maintain the PIPJ in 20° flexion. A synovectomy of the flexor tendons should be done simultaneously, which improves the excursion of the FDP within the flexor sheath. Active mobilization in flexion should be started immediately, and hyperextension blocked using a dorsal splint for 4 to 6 weeks.

Limited passive range of PIPJ motion

The active and passive ranges of motion at the PIPJ are limited in all positions of the MCPJ. This limitation causes a significant disability because the patient is unable to flex the PIPJ to grasp objects. The primary cause of this limited range of motion is adhesion between the central band and dorsally translated conjoint lateral bands over the dorsum of the PIPJ. Over time, a contracture of the dorsal skin over the PIPJ further limits flexion. None of the previously described surgical techniques (eg, tenodesis, joint fusion, and intrinsic release) can by themselves restore motion to the PIPJ. These techniques can be used only when the stiff PIPJ becomes flexible. This flexibility is achieved by releasing the adhesions and soft tissue contractures.

Treatment Adhesions and soft tissue contractures are released by manipulation, with the patient under anesthesia. A surgical release of the joint is considered only in select cases if manipulation is not successful. Patient selection is important because a surgical release needs compliance with a rigorous postoperative therapy regimen, because surgery by itself can lead to increased adhesions and scarring. Before restoring motion at the PIPJ, it is essential to correct any contributing deformity at the MCPJ and the DIPJ and ensure that there are no advanced intra-articular changes at the PIPJ. One should also examine for the presence of digital flexor tenosynovitis, as this may restrict flexor tendon excursion. A patient with RA and flexor tenosynovitis has a good passive range of motion but limited active range of motion, whereas a patient with joint damage has a limitation in both passive motion and active motion.[24]

Technique of manipulation of the PIPJ Manipulation of the PIPJ is preferably done under regional or local anesthesia, as it allows an immediate assessment of the released PIPJ. One aims to manipulate the PIPJ into 80° to 90° of flexion by stretching the soft tissues. This stretching should be done gently to prevent rupture of the attenuated central band and/or fracture of the osteoporotic phalanges. Once adequate passive flexion of the PIPJ is obtained, the patient is asked to actively flex the joint. If the patient is under general anesthesia, traction is applied to the flexor tendons via an incision in the palm to determine if the flexor tendon excursion uses all of the passive PIPJ flexion obtained as a result of joint manipulation.[25] If the patient is unable to do so, one should suspect tenosynovitis of the flexor tendons and perform a flexor tenosynovectomy from a volar approach. Once active and passive range of motion at the PIPJ is established, the patient is started on a therapy program that gradually encourages active range of PIPJ flexion.

Technique of soft tissue release The aim of the soft tissue release is to mobilize the dorsally displaced conjoint lateral bands (**Fig. 7**). A curvilinear incision is made over the dorsum of the proximal phalanx, extending onto the middle phalanx in an oblique fashion. The skin flaps are raised, and the central band is separated from the conjoint lateral bands by 2 longitudinal incisions on both sides of the central band extending from the mid–middle phalanx to mid–proximal phalanx. The conjoint lateral bands are mobilized on either side, and the central band is separated from the dorsum of the proximal phalanx and the underlying joint capsule. The PIPJ is then gently brought into an 80° to 90° flexion. If there is difficulty in getting flexion at the PIPJ, the following maneuvers are done in sequence till passive PIPJ flexion is achieved: (1) resection of the dorsal PIPJ capsule, (2) release of the dorsal portions of the radial and ulnar collateral ligaments from the proximal phalanx, and (3) Z lengthening of the central band.[20] The patient is asked to actively flex the digit, and shifting of the lateral bands volarly on flexion and relocation dorsally on extension should be observed. Only the proximal portion of the incision (till the PIPJ) is closed with the finger in flexion; the distal incision is left to heal spontaneously. The patient is started on a therapy program that gradually encourages range of PIPJ flexion.

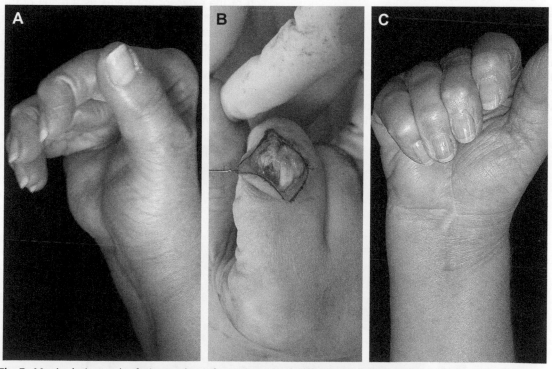

Fig. 7. Manipulation and soft tissue release for correction of stiff swan neck deformities. (*A*) A 66-year-old patient with stiff swan neck deformities of index, long, and ring fingers. (*B*) Longitudinal incision to separate the conjoint lateral band from the central band with manipulation of the PIPJ. (*C*) One-year follow-up showing improvement in range of flexion.

No passive PIPJ motion

In patients with RA and articular damage to the PIPJ surface and/or an unstable dislocated joint, the treatment choices are limited to joint fusion or implant arthroplasty. Although implant arthroplasty seems to be an attractive solution, the authors consider joint fusion to be the more reliable option in patients with RA. The ligamentous support (collateral ligaments, volar plate, and central band) of the PIPJ in RA is usually diseased and does not provide enough stability for implants. This situation is contrary to that seen in osteoarthritis, in which the supporting structures are intact and implant arthroplasty is predictable and reliable. Implant arthroplasty of the PIPJ in RA is limited to the ring and small fingers (index and long fingers need good lateral stability, and flexion is less important) in patients with good adjacent joints (no MCPJ disease), good dorsal skin, intact flexor tendons, and good soft tissue support.[20] This combination of factors is rare in patients with RA and no passive motion at the PIPJ, and arthrodesis of the PIPJ in flexion is the treatment of choice.

BND

BND is characterized by a flexion deformity of the PIPJ with reciprocal extension of the MCPJ and DIPJ (**Fig. 8**).[26]

Pathogenesis

Unlike for SND, there is only 1 etiologic factor for the development of BND in RA, that is, synovitis of the PIPJ.[13,14] The pathologic process begins with the intra-articular proliferation of the synovium in the dorsal synovial pouch, leading to distention

of the capsuloligamentous apparatus and stretching of the central band. The synovium extends as a pannus across the joint and penetrates the bone beneath the collateral ligaments at their attachment to the head of the proximal phalanx. It creates erosions and detachment of the ligaments. The synovium stretches the conjoint lateral bands laterally, breaking through between the central band and the conjoint lateral bands, which, combined with stretching of the central band, leads to a volar displacement of the conjoint lateral bands over the convexity of the phalangeal condyles. The conjoint lateral bands are now volar to the axis of rotation of the PIPJ and become a flexor of the PIPJ instead of the normal role as an extensor. The stretched central band is no longer able to maintain full extension of the PIPJ, and the volarly subluxed conjoint lateral bands maintain persistent PIPJ flexion. Eventually, the head of the proximal phalanx prolapses through the attenuated central slip like a button through a buttonhole (BND) (**Fig. 9**).

The rupture of the central slip means that the interosseous and lumbrical muscles no longer have an insertion into the base of the middle phalanx, and the entire force is now transmitted via the lateral bands to the distal phalanx, with resultant hyperextension of the DIPJ. The proximal migration of the extensor apparatus as a result of the BND allows the pull of the extensor tendon to be concentrated on its insertion into the base of the proximal phalanx, resulting in hyperextension of the MCPJ. Eventually, persistent PIPJ flexion leads to shortening and contracture of the volar plate, collateral ligaments, TRL, and ORLs. The shortening of the ORLs maintains the hyperextension deformity at the DIPJ and limits active flexion

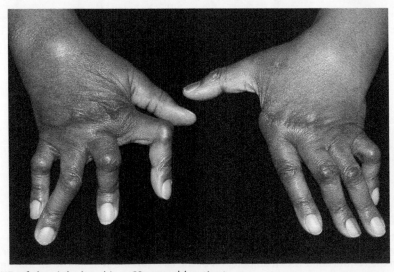

Fig. 8. Classic BND of the right hand in a 69-year-old patient.

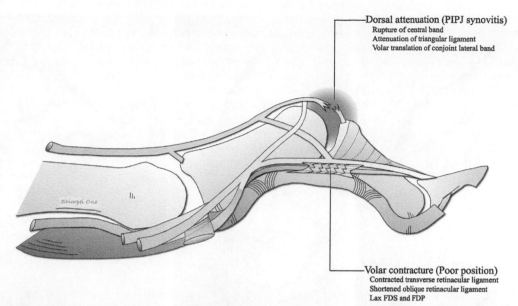

Dorsal attenuation (PIPJ synovitis)
Rupture of central band
Attenuation of triangular ligament
Volar translation of conjoint lateral band

Volar contracture (Poor position)
Contracted transverse retinacular ligament
Shortened oblique retinacular ligament
Lax FDS and FDP

Fig. 9. Pathogenesis of a BND. (*Courtesy of* Dr Shimpei Ono, MD, Tokyo, Japan, s-ono@nms.ac.jp; with permission).

of the DIPJ. The MCPJ hyperextension is exaggerated as a result of the patient trying to compensate for increasing PIPJ flexion deformity. Passive correction of the BND is possible in the early stage, but later on, the BND becomes fixed because of fibrosis and contracture of the capsular structures.[27,28]

Management

The soft tissue reconstruction of rheumatoid BND is unpredictable and often disappointing.[29] Flatt[30] stated that the correction of a BND caused by trauma was difficult and the correction of a BND caused by RA was virtually impossible. A BND is not as functionally disabling as an SND and rarely compromises PIPJ flexion and grip strength (see **Fig. 1B**). One should not trade extension at the PIPJ for a stiff finger and a weak hand. Although this sounds like a pessimistic outlook, the surgical treatment of BND in RA should be tempered with a dose of realism and the surgeon's ability to predictably improve the patient's function. As in the case of an SND, the first step is to determine the passive range of motion at the PIPJ to classify the deformity in 1 of 3 types.

Full passive range of PIPJ motion

In patients with early BND, the PIPJ flexion deformity can be corrected passively as soft tissue contractures have not yet occured. On attempting active PIPJ extension, patients have a 10° to 15° extension lag. One should then examine the PIPJ

for evidence of active synovitis and ascertain if the posture of DIPJ hyperextension becomes better or worse with PIPJ extension. Worsening DIPJ hyperextension with PIPJ extension indicates tightness of the ORL, which is tested using the Haines test.[11] The PIPJ is held extended by the examiner who then assesses the resistance to passive flexion of the DIPJ (**Fig. 10**). Patients with tightness of the ORL have a much greater resistance to passive flexion of the DIPJ, and DIPJ flexion is possible only when the PIPJ is allowed to flex.

Treatment A normal PIPJ in patients with early BND is best treated by splinting the PIPJ in extension. The splint should not extend to the DIPJ, and care must be taken to avoid pressure necrosis of the skin around the PIPJ. The patients should be advised to continue to flex the DIPJ to maintain the lateral bands in a good position. In patients who are unable to flex the DIPJ while the PIPJ is maintained in complete extension because of a tight ORL, an extensor tenotomy is required. If there is PIPJ synovitis that has not responded to oral medications, a single intra-articular injection of corticosteroid can be effective. However, if the synovitis is persistent, synovectomy of the PIPJ is indicated.

Technique of extensor tenotomy The aim of this tenotomy is to divide the terminal tendon insertion such that the contribution of the conjoint lateral bands to the terminal tendon is divided, but the contribution of the ORL to the terminal tendon is

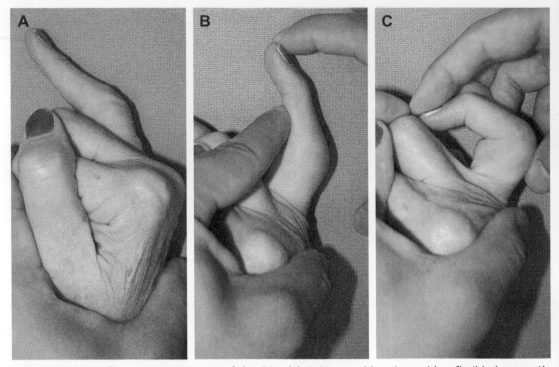

Fig. 10. Haines test for assessing tightness of the ORL. (*A*) A 67-year-old patient with a flexible boutonnière deformity of the right small finger. (*B*) DIPJ flexion is restricted when the PIPJ is maintained in extension. (*C*) Improved range of DIPJ flexion when the PIPJ is allowed to flex.

preserved.[31,32] A longitudinal incision is made over the dorsum of the middle phalanx. The attenuated fibers of the triangular ligament and the volarly displaced conjoint lateral bands are identified over the mid–middle phalanx. The triangular ligament and both the conjoint lateral bands are divided transversely. This division should be done proximal to the attachment of the ORL. A dynamic splint (reverse knuckle bender type) at the PIPJ helps restore proper balance between the joints in the postoperative period. A slight mallet deformity may occur after the tenotomy but is usually well tolerated. If the mallet deformity is significant, the DIPJ is splinted for 4 to 6 weeks in extension. If this splinting does not correct the mallet deformity, a fusion of the DIPJ can be considered.[33]

Limited passive range of PIPJ motion
Patients with limited passive range of PIPJ motion have had the deformity for some period, resulting in soft tissue changes that prevent complete passive correction of the flexion deformity. On attempted active PIPJ extension, these patients have a pronounced extensor lag of 30° to 40° and the MCPJ hyperextension is obvious. Before considering any surgical treatment, patients

should undergo a trial of splinting to try and stretch out the collateral ligaments, volar plate, joint capsule, and volar skin. It is also important to establish that the flexor tendons are intact and functioning and the joint surfaces are smooth on a radiograph. The aim of surgical treatment is to restore extensor force to the PIPJ using local tissues. This restoration is done by excising the attenuated portion of the central band and repairing it and bringing and maintaining the conjoint lateral bands dorsally. In theory, this procedure should correct the BND, but in practice, it is difficult to repair the central band without limiting flexion, which is a high price to pay.[33]

Technique of extensor reconstruction This procedure should be done with the patient under light sedation and digital block so that the surgeon can gauge the tension of the tendon reconstruction, with the patient participating in active finger extension and flexion. A dorsal curvilinear incision is made over the PIPJ, extending from the mid–middle phalanx to mid–proximal phalanx. The incision is curved over the PIPJ so that a skin flap covers the repair of the central band.[33] The central band is divided from the insertion onto the base of the middle phalanx, leaving a cuff of tissue on the middle phalanx to allow repair later. The PIPJ is inspected, and a synovectomy performed, if needed. The central band is separated from the lateral bands proximally, the attenuated distal portion excised (approximately 3–7 mm), and the central band advanced and reattached to the cuff of the tissue at the base of the middle phalanx. Before excising the central band, one must ensure that a repair is possible with the PIPJ flexed to 70° to 80°. A correct judgment of tension is the most critical step in this procedure. Tension can be assessed with an alert patient participating in active finger movement. Next, an incision is made volar to the conjoint lateral bands extending from the mid–proximal phalanx till the mid–middle phalanx on both sides. This incision divides the TRL on either side, but care is taken to preserve the ORL, which runs below the TRL and inserts distally to the terminal tendon (see **Fig. 2**B). The conjoint lateral bands can now be transposed from their displaced volar location to a more dorsal location. The lateral bands are sutured to each other over the mid–proximal phalanx and to the central band over the PIPJ.[34] At this point, one examines if DIPJ flexion is restricted when the PIPJ is extended, and if needed, an extensor tenotomy is performed. The PIPJ is splinted in extension for 4 to 6 weeks to allow the repair of the central band to become strong. The DIPJ is left free, and the patient is encouraged to move it. After 4 to 6 weeks, the static splint is replaced with a dynamic splint during the day and a resting splint at night.

No passive PIPJ motion

No passive PIPJ motion may be either because of a severe soft tissue contracture or a bony ankylosis resulting from erosion of the joint surfaces. A radiograph easily differentiates between these 2 causes. In patients with a severe soft tissue contracture, it is possible to try stretching the soft tissue with a series of plaster casts, then attempt a joint release followed by an extensor reconstruction. However, such an extensive degree of surgery is seldom indicated.[33] The surgical options in these patients and in patients with articular damage are limited to joint fusion or implant arthroplasty. The indications for implant arthroplasty in BND are even more limited when compared with SND because a significant resection of the proximal phalanx is required to seat the implants in the flexed BND, which leads to instability because the collateral ligaments have to be sacrificed.[33] In addition, an extensor reconstruction is needed, which adds to the period before mobilization can be started. The authors' treatment of choice of severe BND is fusion of the PIPJ.

Flexor Tenosynovitis

Synovitis is the hallmark of RA, and in the hand, it involves the synovial lining of the tendon sheath (tenosynovium) and the joint. Flexor tendons are covered by the tenosynovium under the carpal tunnel and in the digital flexor sheath, whereas extensor tendons are covered by tenosynovium only under the extensor retinaculum. The changes in the extensor tendon seen at the interphalangeal joints are caused by the underlying joint synovitis and not tenosynovitis.[17]

Pathogenesis

Synovitis of the hand involves the extensor tendons more frequently than the flexor tendons.[1] As synovitis progresses, the tendon is infiltrated and ultrastructural changes take place in the tendinous tissue, which may include ischemic necrosis, eventually leading to loss of function and rupture without additional mechanical irritation. Three main groups of flexor tenosynovitis can be distinguished: isolated carpal tenosynovitis (20%), palmodigital tenosynovitis (50%), and diffuse tenosynovitis (30%). The index, long, and small fingers are most frequently involved. Rheumatoid nodules are 3 times more frequent in the flexor tendons than in the extensor tendons and are usually confined to the profundus tendon.[35] A flexor tendon rupture in the digital flexor sheath is almost always secondary to infiltrative synovitis and usually involves the FDS at the PIPJ.[36] This is probably because the FDS splits into 2 slips, diminishing the cross-sectional area by half and increasing the surface in contact with the invading synovium in the distal third of the proximal phalanx near the vincula tendinum.[17]

Management

Tenosynovitis can be identified by 3 findings: swelling of the palmar aspect of the digit, discrepancy between active and passive range of motion, and palpable crepitus along the course of the flexor tendon on active and passive flexion of the digit.[24] It can also cause triggering and pain when flexing the finger, loss of active interphalangeal flexion, and an SND in long-standing cases.[37] Tenosynovitis of the flexor tendons is diagnosed by asking the patient to flex the interphalangeal joints while applying some pressure over the tendon proximal to the A1 pulley of the flexor tendon sheath. The patient experiences discomfort, and the examiner notices swelling, grinding, and mild triggering from the hypertrophic synovium going in and out of the flexor tendon sheath. A definitive diagnosis is made when the patient cannot fully flex the interphalangeal joints actively, whereas full passive flexion is possible (**Fig. 11A**).[17] A rheumatoid trigger finger presents as an intermittent somewhat painful triggering on active flexion and extension. Gentle palpation of the flexor sheath during active flexion reveals a nodule moving with the tendon. A trigger finger must be distinguished from the snapping finger that is seen in early SND deformity, when the patient is able to correct the hyperextended position by sudden flexion of the PIPJ. This movement brings the lateral bands below the axis of rotation with a snap.

Treatment

Flexor tenosynovectomy is a safe and effective method for restoring function to rheumatoid patients with flexor tenosynovitis and preventing further complications of flexor tenosynovitis, such as median nerve compression and flexor tendon rupture.[38] The surgical technique for flexor synovectomy requires care to avoid injury to the median nerve, palmar arch, and digital neurovascular bundles. Flexor tenosynovitis may involve multiple sites in the same hand, and it is important to do a complete flexor tenosynovectomy in a single stage. Residual synovitis in an unoperated finger restricts postoperative mobility of the other fingers. The skin incisions must be planned carefully to allow complete access to the disease area without forceful retraction.

Technique of flexor tenosynovectomy

The authors use a Brunner type incision in the fingers and the palm and an extended carpal tunnel incision if access is required more proximally (see **Fig. 11**). The skin flaps are raised carefully, dissecting the neurovascular bundles till the sausage-shaped mass of distended synovium is visualized. The flexor tendons are then delivered into the wound by alternatively pulling on the FDS and the FDP in the gaps between the annular pulleys. The area of tenosynovitis can then be excised from each tendon using a combination of sharp and blunt dissections. Occasionally the tenosynovitis infiltrates into the tendon substance, resulting in a frayed tendon surface. In such cases, the frayed surface should be trimmed. A tendon defect resulting from the excision of a nodule can be closed with a horizontal mattress suture. The slips of the FDS may be infiltrated with tenosynovitis, and the surgeon tempted to excise the FDS tendon. This procedure should be avoided as far as possible because of the progressive nature of the disease. The FDS is the prime flexor of the PIPJ, and excising it may result in an SND. In the presence of intrinsic muscle contracture, the lateral bands should be divided. The bands can be approached by blunt dissection on both sides

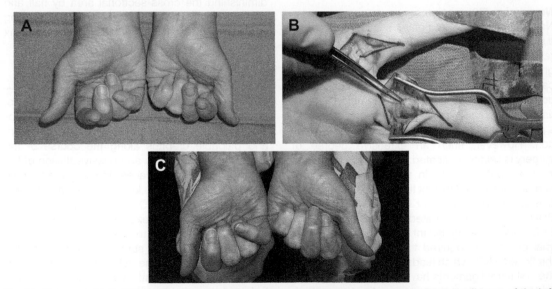

Fig. 11. Rheumatoid digital flexor tenosynovitis. (*A*) A 69-year-old patient with restricted active flexion of the left index, left long, and right index fingers caused by digital flexor tenosynovitis. (*B*) Intraoperative picture showing the appearance of the left long finger before synovectomy and the left index finger after synovectomy. (*C*) Postoperative result at 3 months showing improvement in range of active flexion.

at the base of the proximal phalanx, using the same volar incision. While maintaining the MCPJ in extension, the extensor apparatus is divided from volar to dorsal until the PIPJ can be passively flexed.

The tourniquet is released, and careful hemostasis achieved before loose skin closure with interrupted nylon 4-0 or 5-0 sutures. If the surgery was performed with the patient under local anesthesia or a Bier block, the active range of motion can be visualized before skin closure and any residual diseased areas addressed. A generously padded volar plaster-of-Paris slab extending till the fingertips is applied while maintaining the fingers in an intrinsic plus posture and the wrist in moderate extension. The hand is kept elevated, and gentle mobilization is started in 4 to 7 days.

Treatment of trigger digits

Surgery for trigger fingers in rheumatoid patients consists of flexor tenosynovectomy as outlined earlier and A1 pulley release. Brunner incision should be used in these patients instead of the standard limited palmar incision used for the release of triggers in non-rheumatoid patients. Some investigators recommend resection of 1 slip of the FDS to provide greater space for passage of the FDP instead of A1 pulley release. The release of the A1 pulley contributes toward the MCPJ ulnar drift deformity. This scenario may be true for the index and middle fingers because of the oblique line of pull of the long flexors for these digits, although there are several factors responsible for the ulnar drift deformity.[39]

Treatment of ruptured flexor tendons

The management of a flexor tendon rupture within the digit is difficult, and a flexor tenosynovectomy performed early can prevent this rupture.[38] Rupture of the FDS is frequently overlooked because the patient can still fully flex the finger and the integrity of the FDS tendons is not routinely examined by many surgeons. Palpating the volar aspect of the finger and finding an empty sheath, usually at the level of the proximal phalanx, establishes the level of rupture.

1. Rupture of FDS: One should excise the FDS and carry out tenosynovectomy of the FDP.
2. Rupture of FDP: If the rupture of the FDP has occurred distal to the FDS insertion, it may be possible to advance and repair it because the proximal end is usually caught at the FDS chiasm. However, if repair is not possible or the rupture has occurred proximally, it is better to excise the FDP and do an arthrodesis or tenodesis of the distal interphalangeal joint. Irrespective of what is done for the ruptured

FDP, the most important consideration is to do a complete flexor tenosynovectomy of the FDS to protect it from rupture.
3. Rupture of FDS and FDP: This is a difficult situation, and the chances of obtaining active flexion at the PIPJ are severely limited. Two options are available. One is to carry out flexor tenosynovectomy, insert a silicon rod, and perform a tendon graft procedure at a later date. The other is to fuse the interphalangeal joints and suture one of the long flexors to the base of the proximal phalanx (flexor sheath or bone) to increase the strength of flexion at the MCPJ.

Joint Synovitis

The development and progress of synovitis in the PIPJ has been described previously in the section on SND and BND.[13,14] The role of joint synovectomy (wrist, MCPJ, and interphalangeal joint) in RA has not been established. Whereas it has been shown that recurrence after flexor tenosynovectomy is rare and that tendon ruptures are prevented by tenosynovectomy, there has been no large series of cases that has shown that joint synovectomy can change the course of rheumatoid joint involvement. However, most rheumatoid hand surgeons think that joint synovectomy is useful in certain specific situations. The procedure has a prophylactic value in patients who have a persistent smoldering synovitis, which is never fully controlled by medication and has not yet caused articular erosion. These patients respond to splinting and steroid injections for a few months, and the synovitis flares up again. If left untreated, the synovitis gradually leads to joint destruction. Joint synovectomy is unlikely to be beneficial in the presence of articular erosions; therefore, early identification and excision of persistent synovitis is the basis of a prophylactic synovectomy. The results of soft tissue reconstructive procedures and implant arthroplasty at the PIPJ are unpredictable when compared with those at the wrist and MCPJ. The indications for PIPJ synovectomy are therefore broader, and it can be done even in the presence of some joint destruction. It is a minor procedure resulting in little disability and a short hospitalization, and if it fails, one could then turn to other reconstructive procedures.[38]

Technique of PIPJ synovectomy

A curvilinear dorsal longitudinal skin incision on the dorsum of the PIPJ is used (**Fig. 12**). If the synovial bulging is limited to 1 side, a lateral incision can be used. If a dorsal incision is used, the joint is approached either between the central slip and the lateral band or palmar to the lateral band,

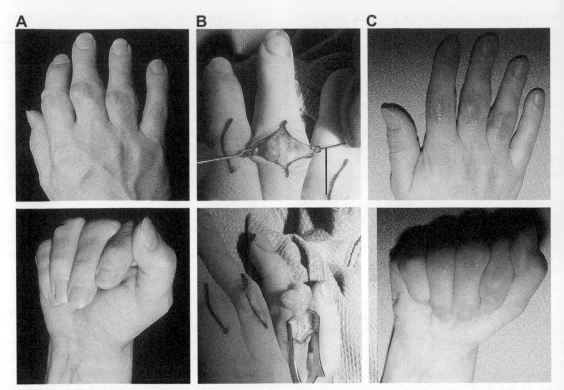

Fig. 12. Technique of synovectomy of the PIPJ. (*A*) A 56-year-old patient with synovitis of the PIPJ of the right index, long, and ring fingers with limited active range of flexion. (*B*) Intraoperative picture showing the appearance of the left long finger before synovectomy and the left ring finger after synovectomy. (*C*) Postoperative result at 3 months showing improvement in range of active flexion.

depending on the location of the disease. If a lateral incision is used, the joint is approached dorsal or palmar to the collateral ligament. Traction on the finger improves the visualization of the joint, and a small rongeur is used to excise the synovium. A small curette is useful to clear the synovial recesses on the palmar and dorsal aspects of the head of the proximal phalanx. The joint is irrigated to wash out any free bits of synovium, and the incision in the extensor mechanism is repaired with 4-0 Vicryl sutures. An early BND may become more pronounced after a synovectomy, and a prophylactic repair should be done immediately. The joint is splinted in extension till the patient is able to perform active extension, and gentle mobilization is started after 4 to 7 days.

SUMMARY

An experienced RA hand surgeon strives to understand the patient's needs and expectations for improvement and attempts to match them with the available surgical options that can predictably improve the patient's function. It is important to collaborate with the referring rheumatologist, who has an intimate knowledge of the patient's overall disease, psychosocial issues, and functional requirements, before deciding whether an operation is needed and what type of procedures should be performed. The correction of digital deformities in RA is akin to putting the icing on the cake or scoring a point after touchdown in American football. The cake or the touchdown itself is more important and refers to the correction of the more proximal deformities (eg, thumb, MCPJ and wrist, extensor tendon reconstruction) that have predictable outcomes and markedly improve the patients' quality of life. This approach creates an environment of trust between the patient, the referring rheumatologist, and the hand surgeon. One can then proceed with the correction of digital deformities. It is also helpful to outline for the patient a sequence of treatment priorities to plan for a long-term relationship. Informing the rheumatologist of the plans helps in their management of the patients before and after surgery. Although the incidence of rheumatoid hand surgery seems to be decreasing, there is still a need for hand surgeons to be involved in the care of the rheumatoid hands because a substantial number of patients may not respond to medications and will still develop hand deformities. It is also uncertain whether these new medications simply delay the inevitable progression of hand and wrist diseases. Hand surgery should remain a partner with rheumatology in the coordinated care of patients whose hand diseases may be treated by the continued innovations in arthroplasty procedures.

REFERENCES

1. Schindele D, Kloss D, Herren D. Options in extensor tendon reconstruction in rheumatoid arthritis. In: Ian Trail MH, editor. Surgery of the rheumatoid hand and wrist. Amsterdam: Elsevier; 2006. p. 94–106.

2. Johnsson PM, Eberhardt K. Hand deformities are important signs of disease severity in patients with early rheumatoid arthritis. Rheumatology 2009; 48(11):1398–401.

3. Eberhardt K, Johnson PM, Rydgren L. The occurrence and significance of hand deformities in early rheumatoid arthritis. Br J Rheumatol 1991;30(3): 211–3.

4. Tubiana R, Toth B. Rheumatoid arthritis: clinical types of deformities and management. In: Wynn Parry CB, editor. Clinics in rheumatic diseases, vol. 5. Philadelphia: WB Saunders; 1984. p. 21–47.

5. Smith RJ. Balance and kinetics of the fingers under normal and pathological conditions. Clin Orthop Relat Res 1974;104:92–111.

6. Doyle J. Hand. In: Doyle J, Botte M, editors. Surgical anatomy of the hand and upper extremity. Philadelphia: Lippincott Williams & Wilkins; 2003. p. 533–667.

7. Yu H, Chase R, Strauch B, editors. Atlas of hand anatomy and clinical implications. St Louis (MO): Mosby; 2003. p. 316–56.

8. Tubiana R, Thomine JM, Mackin E. Movements of the hand and wrist. In: Tubiana R, Thomine JM, Mackin E, editors. Examination of the hand and wrist. St Louis (MO): Mosby; 1996. p. 78–111.

9. Schultz RJ, Furlong J, Storace A. Detailed anatomy of the extensor mechanism at the proximal aspect of the finger. J Hand Surg Am 1981;6:493–8.

10. Thompson J, Littler J, Upton J. The spiral oblique retinacular ligament (SORL). J Hand Surg Am 1978;3:482–7.

11. Haines RW. The extensor apparatus of the finger. J Anat 1951;85:251–9.

12. Heywood AW. The pathogenesis of the rheumatoid swan neck deformity. Hand 1979;11(2):176–83.

13. Harrison SH. Rheumatoid deformities of the proximal interphalangeal joints of the hand. Ann Rheum Dis 1969;28(5):Suppl: 20–2.

14. Harrison SH. The proximal interphalangeal joint in rheumatoid arthritis. Hand 1971;3(2):125–30.

15. Dreyfus JN, Schnitzer TJ. Pathogenesis and differential diagnosis of the swan-neck deformity. Semin Arthritis Rheum 1983;13(2):200–11.

16. Bunnell S, Doherty E, Curtis R. Ischemic contracture, local, in the hand. Plast Reconstr Surg 1946; 3(4):424–33.

17. Lluch A. Examination of the rheumatoid hand and wrist. In: Trail I, Hayton M, editors. Surgery of the rheumatoid hand and wrist. Amsterdam: Elsevier; 2006. p. 9–26.

18. Swanson A. Surgery of the hand in cerebral palsy and swan neck deformity. J Bone Joint Surg Am 1960;42:951–64.

19. Milford L. Sublimis tenodesis technique by Curtis. In: Edmonson A, Crenshaw A, editors. Campbell's operative orthopaedics. 6th edition. St Louis (MO): Mosby; 1980. p. 319.

20. Nalebuff EA, Millender LH. Surgical treatment of the swan neck deformity in rheumatoid arthritis. Orthop Clin North Am 1975;6(3):733–52.

21. Littler J. The finger extensor mechanism. Surg Clin North Am 1967;47:415–32.

22. Zancolli EA, Zancolli E. Surgical rehabilitation of the spastic upper limb in cerebral palsy. In: Lamb DW, editor. The paralysed hand. Edinburgh: Churchill Livingstone; 1987. p. 163–7.

23. Nalebuff EA. The rheumatoid swan neck deformity. Hand Clin 1989;5(2):407–20.

24. Boyer MI, Gelberman RH. Operative correction of swan-neck and boutonniere deformities in the rheumatoid hand. J Am Acad Orthop Surg 1999;7(2): 92–100.

25. Nalebuff E. Surgical treatment of finger deformities in the rheumatoid hand. Surg Clin North Am 1969; 49:833–46.

26. Heywood AW. Correction of the rheumatoid boutonniere deformity. J Bone Joint Surg Am 1969;51: 1309–14.

27. Feldon P, Terrono AL, Nalebuff EA, et al. Rheumatoid arthritis and other connective tissue disorders. In: Green DP, Hotchkiss RN, Pederson WC, et al, editors, In: Greens operative hand surgery, vol. 1. Philadelphia: Elsevier Health Sciences; 2005 . p. 2049–136.

28. Zancolli E. Structural and dynamic bases of hand surgery. Philadelphia: JB Lippincott Company; 1968.

29. Kiefhaber TR, Strickland JW. Soft tissue reconstruction for rheumatoid swan-neck and boutonniere deformities: long-term results. J Hand Surg Am 1993;18(6):984–9.

30. Flatt A. Intra-articular thio-tepa in rheumatoid disease of the hands. Rheumatism 1960;18:70–3.

31. Dolphin J. Extensor tenotomy for chronic boutonniere deformity of the finger: report of two cases. J Bone Joint Surg Am 1965;47:161–4.

32. Fowler S. The hand in rheumatoid arthritis. Am Surg 1963;29:403–4.

33. Nalebuff EA, Millender LH. Surgical treatment of the boutonniere deformity in rheumatoid arthritis. Orthop Clin North Am 1975;6(3):753–63.

34. Urbaniak J, Hayes M. Chronic boutonniere deformity—an anatomic reconstruction. J Hand Surg Am 1981;6(4):379–83.

35. Saffar P. Flexor tendon synovectomy in rheumatoid arthritis. In: Trail I, Hayton M, editors. Surgery of the rheumatoid hand and wrist. Amsterdam: Elsevier; 2006. p. 107–17.

36. Ertol AN, Millender LH, Nalebuff EA, et al. Flexor tendon ruptures in patients with rheumatoid arthritis. J Hand Surg Am 1988;13(6):860–6.

37. Lluch A. The treatment of finger joint deformities in rheumatoid arthritis. In: Allieu Y, editor. The rheumatoid hand and wrist. Paris: Expansion Scientifique Publications; 1998. p. 85–104.

38. Millender LH, Nalebuff EA. Preventive surgery — tenosynovectomy and synovectomy. Orthop Clin North Am 1975;6(3):765–92.

39. Ferlic DC, Clayton ML. Flexor tenosynovectomy in the rheumatoid finger. J Hand Surg Am 1978;3:364–7.

Tendon Reconstruction for the Rheumatoid Hand

Stephan F. Schindele, MD*, Daniel B. Herren, MD,
Beat R. Simmen, MD

KEYWORDS

- Rheumatoid arthritis • Tendon rupture
- Tendon reconstruction • Tendon graft • Tendon transfer

EXTENSOR TENDONS

Rheumatoid arthritis is essentially a disease of the synovial membranes, with all its consequences. The tendon sheaths lined with synovial tissue that surround the tendons in the region of the hand and wrist may be involved in the rheumatoid process as well as the synovial membranes of the joints. Tenosynovitis in the context of rheumatoid arthritis occurs frequently and may become manifest months before signs of joint involvement are identified.[1–3]

Although there has been an awareness of spontaneous tendon rupture for a long time, it was Vaughan-Jackson[4] who in 1948 drew attention to the importance of tendinous alterations with reference to 2 cases of spontaneous rupture of the extensor tendons at the level of the distal radioulnar joint (DRUJ). This report was followed by an increasing number of reports on the pathology of the tendons in rheumatoid arthritis. Investigations undertaken by Kellgern and Ball[5] in 1950 revealed that the tendons were affected by typical alterations in more than 50% of cases.

Synovitic involvement of the extensor tendons have been observed more frequently than that of the flexor tendons in the hand. Mannsat[6] diagnosed dorsal tenosynovitis in 30% of his patients as opposed to palmar in only 22%. It is particularly noticeable that the abductor pollicis longus and extensor pollicis brevis (EPB) were rarely affected in the region of the first tendon compartment.

The clinical picture of rheumatoid tenosynovitis depends on its localization. In most of the cases, tenosynovitis causes pain whereby spontaneous tendon rupture can be an entirely painless event. Primarily, synovitis tends only to affect the mobile tissue of the tendon sheath. During the course of the disease, the tendon is infiltrated, and ultrastructural changes take place in the tendinous tissue, which may include ischemic necrosis, and may lead to loss of function and eventually rupture even without additional mechanical irritation.[7] Progress has clearly been made in the treatment of rheumatoid arthritis in recent years because of the further development and improvement of remedial medication. Drug therapy has had a particularly positive effect on the treatment of tenosynovitis so that this condition is not as prevalent and spontaneous tendon rupture has become less common.

Today, the main cause of spontaneous rupture of the extensor tendons at the wrist is attrition of the tendons over bony spurs. This type of attrition is seen predominantly in the region of the ulnar head and Lister tubercle. The latter forms a bony deflection sheave for the extensor pollicis longus (EPL) tendon and is subject to mechanical load accordingly.

The authors have nothing to disclose.
Department of Upper Extremity and Handsurgery, Schulthess Clinic, Lengghalde 2, CH–8008 Zurich, Switzerland
* Corresponding author.
E-mail address: stephan.schindele@kws.ch

Hand Clin 27 (2011) 105–113
doi:10.1016/j.hcl.2010.10.004

The head of the ulna, adjacent to which lies the ulnar extensor digitorum tendons, dislocates dorsally if there is instability of the DRUJ and supination deformity of the carpus and likewise forms a deflection sheave for the adjacent tendons. Surgical revision aims to eliminate the cause of rupture. As a rule, rupture has been caused by attrition of the tendon over the dorsally protruding ulnar head (caput ulnae syndrome) (**Fig. 1**). In most cases, resection of the head of the distal ulna alone is sufficient (Darrach procedure). If radiology suggests possible radiocarpal instability, according to Simmen classification, arthrodesis of the DRUJ (Sauve-Kapandji procedure) should be preferred combined with radiocarpal partial arthrodesis, if required.[8,9]

A prerequisite for an adequate function of tendon reconstruction is a decent joint function. In rheumatoid patients, it is mandatory to assess joint function preoperatively. In patients with significant impaired joint function, additional joint reconstruction should be planned at the same time as tendon reconstruction.

Diagnosis

Spontaneous extensor tendon ruptures are usually painless and become apparent after minor injury or during normal use of the hand. The initial presentation is sudden loss of ability to extend one or more fingers (**Fig. 2**). Patients with rheumatoid arthritis are used to functional limitations and disabilities associated with their illness. They usually seek medical advice only if the loss of function becomes relevant. Especially isolated ruptures of the extensor digiti quinti (EDQ) and the EPL tendons cause very slight functional loss and are often overlooked and masked by other more severe deformities.

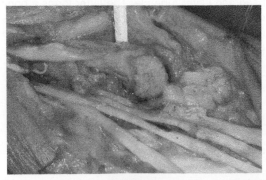

Fig. 1. Caput ulnae syndrome: dorsally protruding ulna head with sharp bony edges causes extensor tendon ruptures of EDQ and EDC4+5.

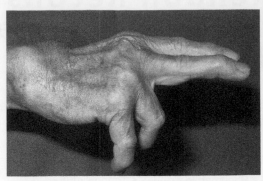

Fig. 2. Clinical presentation of EDQ and EDC4+5 rupture with synovitis and dorsal dislocation of the ulna head (caput ulnae syndrome).

Technique of Extensor Tendon Reconstruction

Rupture of EPL tendon

Rupture of the EPL tendon in the context of rheumatoid arthritis is a frequent event. However, the functional loss caused by it can differ greatly and depend essentially on the functionality of the intact EPB and the status of the joints of the thumb. EPL rupture is often characterized by active functional loss at the interphalangeal (IP) joint, but more frequently, there is a reduction of extension strength and extension arc at the metacarpophalangeal (MCP) joint. Normally, the EPB tendon is too weak to compensate for full extension ability of the MCP joint. In addition, the intrinsic muscles also contribute to the extension of the IP joint.

Restoration of EPL function is recommended if there is severe functional disability. End-to-end suture is generally no longer possible, even immediately after rupture, and this applies to all spontaneous rheumatic ruptures. Tendon grafts that have been woven through tissue altered by inflammatory processes tend to adhere and, therefore, are not necessarily recommended for the repair of ruptured extensor tendons in the rheumatoid hand. Nevertheless, as long as a contractile muscle is present, reconstruction of the EPL by tendon grafting can lead to a good clinical outcome.

The treatment of choice to restore EPL function is generally tendon transfer. The most frequently used donors are the musculo-tendon units of the extensor indicis proprius (EIP) or, less often, the tendons of the extensor carpi radialis longus (ECRL) or EDQ. Nalebuff and colleagues[10] advocate EIP transfer, because the EIP tendon can be released at the MCP joint level, without any apparent functional loss for this joint. Even more surprising is that the patient does not lose the ability to extend the index finger independently from the other long fingers. Strength and amplitude of the EIP are almost identical to those of the EPL.[11,12]

If there is rupture of at least 2 ulnar extensor tendons in addition to EPL rupture, then the EIP is less available, because it is required for reconstruction of the ulnar tendons. In these cases, the reconstruction technique of choice will be a palmaris longus graft. If the palmaris longus is missing, a strip of ECRL, plantaris, or extensor tendon of the 4th toe may serve as graft. However, tendon grafting is only appropriate for relatively fresh ruptures where there is good contractility of the proximal musculo-tendon unit.

If the rupture is present for more than 3 months, transfer of EPL to the EPB will be appropriate.[13] In

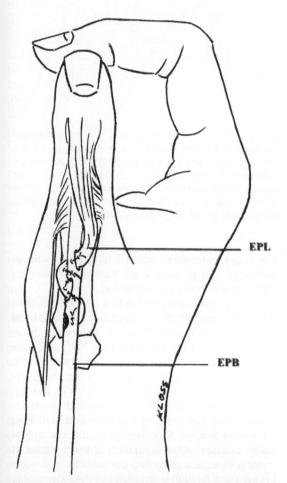

Fig. 3. Restoration of IP extension in the thumb can be achieved by transferring the EPL to the EPB over the thumb metacarpal. (*From* Schindele S, Kloss D, Herren D. Options in extensor tendon reconstruction in rheumatoid arthritis. FESSH Instructional Course Book, International Congress Series 1295 (2006) 94–106; with permission.)

this procedure, the distal stump of the EPL is weaving in the EPB over the thumb metacarpal (**Fig. 3**). Clinically, only simultaneous extension of the interphalangeal and MCP joints is regained, but this leads only to a slight functional restriction.

Rupture of the long-finger extensor tendons

Rupture of a single long-finger extensor can affect any finger, but the small finger is affected most frequently. The extent of active extension loss at the MCP joint of the small finger depends on whether only the EDQ or both the EDQ and the extensor digitorum conununis (EDC) of the little finger are ruptured. Isolated rupture of the EDQ tends to cause only slight loss of active extension at the MCP joint and almost always remains unnoticed. The relevant function test requires the patient to stretch the small finger with the fist clenched. This stretching of the small finger blocks the action of the EDC to the little finger. An extension deficit of 30° to 40° will be observed if the EDQ is dysfunctional.

Reconstruction of the EDQ tendon is most easily achieved by end-to-side suture of the distal tendon stump to the adjacent tendons of EDC-little or EDC-ring. Correct initial tension is essential for the result. The tenodesis effect tested intraoperatively during movement of the wrist must allow all 4 fingers to be moved simultaneously.

Another possibility for primary tendon transfer is to place the EIP tendon into the tendon stump of the small finger extensors (EDQ/EDC5). Before planning this procedure, the integrity of EDC-index must be assessed so that the extension of the index finger is not jeopardized. The EIP tendon is located on the ulnar side of the EDC-index tendon and both pass through the 4th extensor compartment with the EDC tendons. Because the muscle belly is situated very distally, it can easily be differentiated from the EDC tendons. The favorable technique to perform the tendon transfer is the weaving technique described by Pulvertaft. Three or more tendon passages allow secure fixation of the transferred tendon. It is important to maintain adequate tension to have a good functional result. Intraoperatively, the small finger should achieve somewhat greater extension at the MCP joint than the ring finger. Complete passive fist closure should be possible with the wrist in 30° to 40° extension.

If more than one spontaneous extensor tendon rupture is found, for example in the small finger and the long finger, side-to-side suture of both distal tendon stumps to the intact neighbor tendon can be performed. On the one hand, the strength of the middle finger is hardly sufficient to achieve full extension of the 3 ulnar-sided fingers, whereas on the other hand, the stump of the small finger tendon is often too short to reach the long finger for this reconstruction technique.

Tendon grafting or EIP transfer can be performed to restore extension to the small finger, and the ring finger distal tendon stump can be sutured to the long finger in an end-to-side fashion (**Fig. 4**).

If there are 3 or more extensor tendon ruptures, a side-to-side repair to the intact radial communis tendon together with an EIP tendon transfer weaving in 2 distal tendon stumps can be performed (**Fig. 5**).

EIP tendon transfer is the most common procedure, but transfer of the wrist extensors has also been described. However, transfer of the extensor carpi ulnaris is a less appropriate, because this tendon is an important wrist stabilizer and its removal would favor the radial rotation of the wrist observed in rheumatoid patients. Moreover, the wrist extensors have less gliding amplitude than

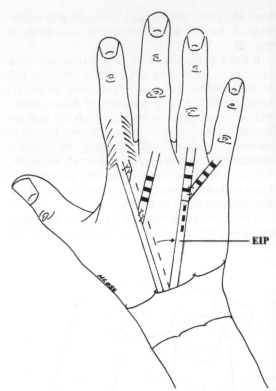

Fig. 5. Restoration of little, ring, and middle finger extensions by end-to-side suture technique of the EDC3 to EDC2 and EIP transfer to EDQ/EDC4/5. (*From* Schindele S, Kloss D, Herren D. Options in extensor tendon reconstruction in rheumatoid arthritis. FESSH Instructional Course Book, International Congress Series 1295 (2006) 94–106; with permission.)

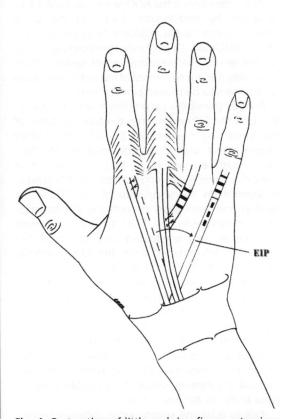

Fig. 4. Restoration of little and ring finger extensions by end-to-side suture technique of the EDC4 to EDC3 and EIP transfer to EDQ. (*From* Schindele S, Kloss D, Herren D. Options in extensor tendon reconstruction in rheumatoid arthritis. FESSH Instructional Course Book, International Congress Series 1295 (2006) 94–106; with permission.)

the finger extensors, which limits the functional outcome, and an insufficient flexion or extension after transfer has to be accepted.

Although reconstruction with a free tendon graft may be problematic because of the risk of secondary adhesions,[14] good outcomes have been described for this technique.[15–17] Possible donors for tendon graft are not only the palmaris longus and strips of ECRL or ECRB but also plantaris tendon and the extensor tendon of the 4th toe. Intraoperatively, the grafts should be maintained under relatively high tension and stabilized by weave sutures to compensate for the anticipated postoperative elongation of the muscles. If muscle fibrosis with limited contractility is already present and tension is too high but the extensibility of the fingers is good, functional restriction may result due to loss of finger flexion. Because atrophy and muscle fibrosis start soon after the rupture, the time to graft reconstruction should not exceed 12 to 20 weeks after the tendon laceration.[17,18] Nakamura and Katsuki,[18] therefore, recommend that tendon grafting should not be performed if there is a contracted proximal musculo-tendon unit and if passive excursion of less than 2 cm is present.

In case of rupture of all finger extensors, a bridge graft may be useful to repair all 4 long-finger extensors. Here, the same rules apply as outlined earlier with regard to time of operation and donor tendons. While reconstructing such mass ruptures, it should be taken into consideration that the likelihood of tendon insufficiency and tendon adhesions also increases with an increase in the number of grafted tendons.

Obviously, when choosing a tendon transfer, the only tendons that are available are from the volar side. A similar technique as described by Boyes[19] for the reconstruction in radial nerve palsy can be used in these patients. The flexor digitorum superficialis (FDS) tendons of the ring and middle fingers are detached from the distal palm and passed through the interosseous membrane from the flexor to the extensor side of the hand. Nalebuff and Patel[20] modified this technique in the way that the superficialis tendon is not threaded through the interosseous membrane but is passed radially around the radius in a dorsal direction (**Fig. 6**). Ulnar-sided transfer is also possible; however, it is not recommended, because it might provoke ulnar drift of the wrist and fingers.

With this technique, up to 3 extensor tendons can be motorized by 1 superficialis tendon. However, if there is rupture of all the extensor tendons, then transfer of 2 superficialis tendons is required. Extension of the ring and long fingers can be restored with the FDS-ring tendon, and extension of the index and middle fingers can be reconstructed with the FDS-long tendon. It is important that the integrity of the relevant profundus tendons is assessed before detachment to ensure that excision will not lead to finger flexion insufficiency. **Table 1** gives an overview of the most recommended procedures.

Postoperative care after extensor tendon reconstruction

Until swelling and pain are controlled, a volar splint with the wrist in 30° to 40° of extension and the MCP joints in slight flexion of 10° to 20° is recommended. Then gentle active motion of the proximal interphalangeal and distal interphalangeal joints is started, whereas the wrist and the MCP joints are still immobilized for 3 to 4 weeks. Because impairment of finger flexion is functionally more limiting than a slight extension lag, it is important to encourage full finger flexion during that rehabilitation phase. Although dynamic splints have the theoretical potential to prevent adhesions, they

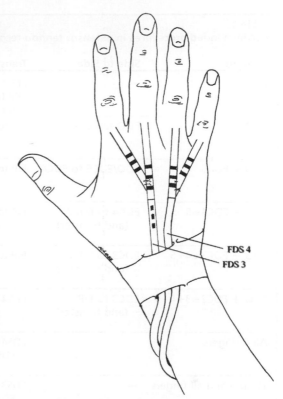

Fig. 6. Restoration of all long-finger extensors by radially passed tendon transfer of the FDS3 to index and middle finger and FDS4 to ring and little finger extensor stumps. (*From* Schindele S, Kloss D, Herren D. Options in extensor tendon reconstruction in rheumatoid arthritis. FESSH Instructional Course Book, International Congress Series 1295 (2006) 94–106; with permission.)

are not used on a routine basis. However, the application of a dynamic splint might be considered in cases with multiple bridge grafts to prevent tendon adhesions and to protect the double-sided weave sutures (**Fig. 7**).

FLEXOR TENDONS

Proliferative synovitis affects the flexor tendons by infiltration, causes nodule formation, changes their ultrastructure, and eventually leads to spontaneous rupture, similar as what has been described in the extensor tendons. The 2 most common sites of tendon sheath and direct tendon involvement by synovitis are the volar side of the wrist and the flexor tendons in the digital canal.

Ertel and colleagues'[21,22] report on 115 flexor tendon ruptures, the majority of these cases were found at the level of the wrist. Two-thirds of these tendon lacerations were associated with bony spurs, the rest showed synovial infiltration

Table 1
Recommended procedures in extensor tendon reconstruction in rheumatoid arthritis

Rupture	Side to Side	Transfer	Graft
EPL	—	EIP EPB (if EIP is needed for ulnar fingers)	Palmaris longus, ECRL/ECRB (only a strip) Extensor tendon of the 4th toe
EDQ	EDQ to EDC4/5	EIP to EDQ	Palmaris longus, ECRL/ECRB (only a strip) Extensor tendon of the 4th toe
EDQ + EDC5	EDQ/EDC5 to EDC4	EIP to EDQ/EDC5	Palmaris longus, ECRL/ECRB (only a strip) Extensor tendon of the 4th toe
EDQ + EDC4+5	EDC4 to EDC3 (and transfer)	EIP to EDQ/EDC5	Palmaris longus, ECRL/ECRB (only a strip) Extensor tendon of the 4th toe
EDQ + EDC3+4+5	EDC3 to EDC2 (and transfer)	EIP to EDQ/EDC4	Palmaris longus, ECRL/ECRB (only a strip) Extensor tendon of the 4th toe
EDQ + EDC2+3+4+5	EDC3 to EIP (and transfer)	FDS4 to EDQ/EDC4	Palmaris longus, ECRL/ECRB (only a strip) Extensor tendon of the 4th toe
All 4 fingers	—	FDS4 to EDQ/EDC4 and FDS3 to EDC2+3/EIP	Palmaris longus ECRL/ECRB (only a strip) Extensor tendon of the 4th toe
Thumb and all fingers	—	FDS3 to EPL/EIP and FDS4 to EDC3-5	—

alone. Only 20% of tendon ruptures were observed in the digital canal.

Multiple flexor tendon ruptures, as an end point of the disease in some patients, are virtually untreatable and provide almost total loss of function of the hand. Fortunately, only the minority of patients suffers rupture of the flexor tendons, but the local effect of proliferative synovitis, either acute or chronic, impairs the grasping function of the hand significantly. The treatment of this condition therefore requires high priority.

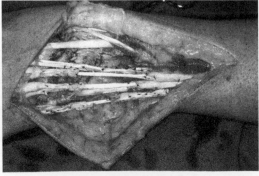

Fig. 7. Left hand: tendon reconstruction of all 4 fingers by grafting.

Early tenosynovectomy has the potential to prevent flexor tendon ruptures and should therefore be the cornerstone of treatment. Meticulous physical examination of the flexor tendons is crucial, because early synovial inflammation may be almost pain free. The presence of trigger fingers is often the earliest sign of the disease, and although steroid injection often relieves the symptoms, a number of patients continue to have acute synovitis.

Once the tendon rupture has occurred, immediate diagnostic workup is needed together with early treatment to prevent further ruptures. Rupture of an isolated tendon is more common than multiple tendon rupture. The most vulnerable tendon is the flexor pollicis longus (FPL). This tendon crosses the scaphotrapezial joint where attrition leads to fraying of the tendon. In addition, local synovitis and joint involvement of other carpal joints can create sharp bony spikes, which weaken the flexor tendons further. The flexor digitorum profundus of the index finger and, to a lesser degree, those of the middle finger are also at risk. There are rare cases in which either extreme dorsal extension[23] or extreme volar flexion[24] of the lunate can cause flexor tendon ruptures.

Diagnosis

Synovitis of the flexor tendons within the palm of the hand and the palmar aspect of the fingers can easily be detected by clinical examination. Swelling, nodules, and crepitus when flexing the finger joints suggest inflammatory tenosynovitis. The presence of trigger fingers may be the first sign of rheumatoid disease. At the level of the wrist, flexor tendon synovitis may be difficult to detect. However, in rheumatoid patients with symptoms of carpal tunnel syndrome, flexor tendon synovitis is to be expected. A late sign of flexor tenosynovitis within the carpal canal can be a spontaneous rupture of the FPL, with the sudden inability to actively flex the IP joint of the thumb.

Although the presence of tenosynovitis can be clinically diagnosed, the extent of the synovitis, its severity, the presence of nodules, and the state of the tendons should be worked up either by ultrasonography or by magnetic resonance imaging (MRI). The presence of tenosynovitis in the MRI of the wrist may even be an early predictor of rheumatoid arthritis.[25]

Tenosynovectomy of Flexor Tendons

Inability to fully flex a finger or symptoms of a trigger finger is an early sign of flexor tendon involvement in patients suffering from rheumatoid arthritis. Local corticosteroid injections may often be curative in these cases. However, despite this therapy, including adequate medical treatment, there are a number of patients who continue to have synovial inflammation. If after a period of 3 to 6 months no improvement is observed when the normal onset of the therapeutic effect of modern drug therapy is to be expected, surgical synovectomy is indicated.

The complexity of performing flexor tendon synovectomy should not be underestimated. Usually the presence of synovitis at the level of the neck of the fibrous A1 pulley would require simple decompression. However, de Jager and colleagues[26] have shown that extensive release of the A1 pulley in patients with rheumatoid arthritis results in an increased palmar subluxation of the MCP joint. Synovectomy should therefore be performed with sharp dissection of the synovitis from the tendon, and if no free tendon gliding is achieved, a minimal release of the A1 pulley is required. Through several pulley windows along the whole tendon sheet, tenosynovectomy can be performed without violating the stability of the flexor tendon. In cases of more extensive synovial proliferation, especially in the acute phase of the disease, increased exposure is required.

Occasionally, it is necessary to explore the flexor tendons from proximal to the wrist up to the level of the distal IP joint in each finger. This is a major surgical intervention, and the rehabilitation process has to be monitored closely during the first postoperative weeks. Extensive debridement of the tendon includes the risk of delayed tendon rupture, especially in vigorous, active therapy programs. A good balance between aggressive remobilization and adequate time for healing is needed, and this requires a good communication between the surgeon and the therapist (**Figs. 8 and 9**).

Isolated Flexor Tendon Rupture

Isolated flexor tendon rupture is more common than multiple tendon lacerations. As outlined, the rupture occurs by far more frequently at the level of the wrist compared with lesions in the digital canal. Early diagnosis is mandatory in order to prevent tendon damage. Rupture is easily possible in the palm and the fingers but is more challenging at the level of the volar wrist. In addition, tenosynovitis of the flexor tendons in the carpal canal hardly produces functional impairment up to the moment when pain-free tendon rupture occurs.

Rupture of the FPL Tendon

The FPL tendon is most vulnerable to fraying or attrition rupture as it crosses the scaphotrapezial joint. Rheumatoid joint disease and local synovitis can create sharp spikes of bone against which the tendon abrades and finally ruptures during use. The deep flexor to the index finger and, less frequently, to the long finger are also at risk at this specific anatomic site.

Rupture of the FPL means a serious functional impairment for the thumb and typically requires

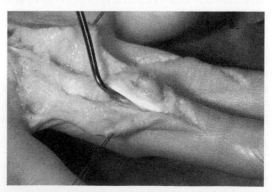

Fig. 8. Typical flexor tendon nodule at the level of the A3 pulley.

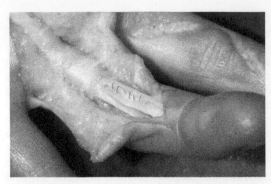

Fig. 9. After removal of the nodule and tendon repair.

treatment. It is important to distinguish 2 different goals in treatment:

Restoration of thumb function
Prevention of further tendon ruptures, especially the flexor digitorum profundus to the index.

So beside any reconstruction for the missing tendon, exploration of the carpal canal is mandatory to detect impending rupture of other flexor tendons and removal of any bony erosion.

Particularly in the thumb, single-stage reconstruction with a tendon graft, usually taken from the palmaris longus tendon or the flexor carpi radialis tendon, is most successful. As in any other tendon reconstruction procedure, it must be assured that the musculo-tendon unit is still functional and an adequate tendon excursion is present.

In the case of a long-standing rupture and doubtful muscle function, a tendon transfer might be more advisable. Typically, the superficial flexor tendon of the ring finger is used for the reconstruction of the thumb flexion. This is best performed by an end-to-end suture in the technique described for the extensor tendon reconstruction. In acute ruptures of the FPL, tendon lengthening at the musculotendinous junction and direct end-to-end suture after adequate debridement may also be considered.

Alternatively, the IP joint of the thumb may be stabilized by fusion. In these cases, it is mandatory to have a functioning MCP joint. In addition, acceptable muscle strength of the intrinsic thumb muscle must be present to give a satisfactory pinch force.

Multiple Tendon Ruptures

Multiple flexor tendon ruptures are very difficult to treat but on the other hand mean an almost total loss of function. Again, early diagnosis is mandatory to prevent such a devastating situation.

Reconstruction of hands with multiple flexor tendon ruptures incorporates all techniques of tendon repair, including grafting, transfer of sublimis to profundus flexor tendons, and splitting profundus tendons to power more than one finger.

In desperate situations with aggressive disease and limited functional requirements, fusion of the IP joints may provide at least some grasping function. But acceptable power should be present in the intrinsic musculature to give a satisfactory grip function.

Fractional Flexor Tendon Lengthening for Advanced MCP Flexion Contracture in Rheumatoid Hands

Rheumatoid arthritis often produces the characteristic MCP joint deformities of palmar dislocation and ulnar deviation. Surgical reconstruction typically includes arthroplasty and soft tissue rebalancing. Associated MCP joint flexion contracture is usually mild and easily corrected by metacarpal head excision alone. In patients suffering from systemic lupus erythematosus, the articular surface is often well preserved, despite the severe flexion contracture. In these cases, it is possible to correct the deformity by combined MCP joint volar capsulotomy, intrinsic release, and metacarpal shortening osteotomy.[27] However, the authors' personal experience with this type of shortening osteotomy in patients with classic rheumatoid arthritis was disappointing.[28]

Al-Ahaideb and colleagues[29] have described a group of patients suffering from mixed connective tissue disease with severe fixed flexion contracture and destroyed MCP joints. In these patients, conventional MCP arthroplasty alone was insufficient to correct the deformity. Instead of correcting the contracture by additional resection of the metacarpal neck and shaft, fractional lengthening of the flexor tendons was advocated. This was achieved by individual lengthening of the superficial flexor tendons by intramuscular transverse tenotomy and circumferential fasciotomy as described by Zancolli and colleagues[30] and Le Viet.[31] In some severe contractures, some or all of the profundus tendons were also lengthened. For this small subgroup of patients with rheumatoid arthritis with mixed connective tissue disease and severe flexion contractures, fractional flexor tendon lengthening may be a reasonable adjunctive procedure to MCP arthroplasty.

ACKNOWLEDGMENTS

The authors wish to thank Danni Jakubietz-Kloss, MD, for the schematic drawings of tendon transfer procedures.

REFERENCES

1. Jakobs JH, Hess EV, Beswick IP. Rheumatoid arthritis presenting as tenosynovitis. J Bone Joint Surg Br 1957;39:288–92.
2. Kay AGL. Natural history of synovial hypertrophy in the rheumatoid hand. Ann Rheum Dis 1971;30:98–102.
3. Nalebuff EA, Potter TA. Rheumatoid involvement of tendon and tendon sheaths in the hand. Clin Orthop 1968;59:147–59.
4. Vaughan-Jackson OJ. Rupture of extensor tendons by attrition at the inferior radio-ulnar joint. Report of two cases. J Bone Joint Surg Br 1948;30:528–30.
5. Kellgern JH, Ball J. Tendon lesions in rheumatoid arthritis. A clinical-pathological study. Ann Rheum Dis 1950;9:46–65.
6. Mannsat M. La main rheumatoide [dissertation]. Touluse (France); 1970.
7. Neurath MF, Stofft E. Ultrastructure of the long flexor and extensor tendons of the hand in rheumatic tenosynovitis. Handchir Mikrochir Plast Chir 1992;24:159–64.
8. Simmen BR, Huber H. [The wrist joint in chronic polyarthritis–a new classification based on the type of destruction in relation to the natural course and the consequences for surgical therapy]. Handchir Mikrochir Plast Chir 1994;26(4):182–9 [in German].
9. Flury MP, Herren DB, Simmen BR. Rheumatoid arthritis of the wrist. Classification related to the natural course. Clin Orthop 1999;366:72–7.
10. Nalebuff EA, Feldo PG, Millender LH. Rheumatoid arthritis in the hand and wrist. In: Green DP, editor. Operative hand surgery. New York: Churchill Livingstone; 1988. p. 1667–77.
11. Browne EZ, Teague MA, Snyder TC. Prevention of extensor lag after indicis proprius tendon transfer. J Hand Surg 1979;4:168–72.
12. Moore JR, Weiland AJ, Valdata L. Independent index extension after extensor indicis proprius transfer. J Hand Surg Am 1987;12:232–6.
13. Harrison S, Swannell AJ, Ansel BM. Repair of extensor pollicis longus using extensor pollicis brevis in rheumatoid arthritis. Ann Rheum Dis 1972;31:490–2.
14. Flatt AE, editor. The care of rheumatoid hand. 3rd edition. St Louis: CV Mosby Company; 1974. p. 114.
15. Bora FW Jr, Osterman AL, Thomas VJ, et al. The treatment of ruptures of multiple extensor tendons at wrist level by a free tendon graft in the rheumatoid patient. J Hand Surg Am 1987;12:1038–40.
16. Minami M, Kato S, Yamazaki J, et al. Tendon ruptures in the rheumatoid hand. In: Vastamäki M, editor. Current trends in hand surgery. Amsterdam: Elsevier Science B V; 1995. p. 515–21.
17. Mountney J, Blundell CM, McArthur P, et al. Free tendon interposition grafting for the repair of ruptured extensor tendons in the rheumatoid hand. J Hand Surg Br 1998;23:662–5.
18. Nakamura S, Katsuki M. Tendon grafting for extensor tendon ruptures of fingers in rheumatoid hands. J Hand Surg Br 2002;27(4):326–8.
19. Boyes JH. Bunnell's surgery of the hand. 5th edition. Philadelphia: Lippincott; 1970. p. 419.
20. Nalebuff EA, Patel MR. Flexor digitorum sublimis transfer for multiple extensor tendon ruptures in rheumatoid arthritis. Plast Reconstr Surg 1973;52:530–3.
21. Ertel AN, Millender LH, Nalebuff E, et al. Flexor tendon ruptures in patients with rheumatoid arthritis. J Hand Surg Am 1988;13:860–6.
22. Ertel AN. Flexor tendon ruptures in rheumatoid arthritis. Hand Clin 1989;5:177–90.
23. Zangger P, Simmen BR. Spontaneous ruptures of flexor tendons secondary to extreme DISI deformity of the lunate in a rheumatoid wrist. A case report. Ann Chir Main Memb Super 1993;12(4):250–6.
24. Baer W, Dumont CE. Mechanical wearing down of flexor tendons in rheumatoid arthritis as a result of extreme volar-flexed intercalated segment instability. Scand J Plast Reconstr Surg Hand Surg 2002;36(3):189–91.
25. Eshed I, Feist E, Althoff CE, et al. Tenosynovitis of the flexor tendons of the hand detected by MRI: an early indicator of rheumatoid arthritis. Rheumatology 2009;48:887–91.
26. de Jager LT, Jaffe R, Learmonth ID, et al. The A1 pulley in rheumatoid flexor tenosynovectomy. To retain or to divide? J Hand Surg Br 1994;19(2):202–4.
27. Hastings DE, Evans JA. The lupus hand: a new surgical approach. J Hand Surg 1978;5:179–83.
28. Herren DB, Simmen BR. Shortening osteotomy for treatment of metacarpophalangeal joint deformity. Clin Orthop Relat Res 2002;394:186–91.
29. Al-Ahaideb A, Drosdowech DS, Pichora DR. Fractional flexor tendon lengthening for advanced metacarophalangeal flexion contracture in rheumatoid hands. J Hand Surg Am 2006;31:1690–3.
30. Zancolli EA, Goldner LJ, Swanson AB. Surgery of the spastic hand in cerebral palsy: report of the Committee on Spastic Hand Evaluation (International Federation of Societies for Surgery of the Hand). J Hand Surg 1983;8:766–72.
31. Le Viet D. Flexor tendon lengthening by tenotomy at the musculotendinous junction. Ann Plast Surg 1986;17:239–46.

Outcomes Research in Rheumatoid Arthritis

Jennifer F. Waljee, MD, MS, Kevin C. Chung, MD, MS*

KEYWORDS

- Rheumatoid arthritis • Hand surgery • Patient outcomes
- Methodology

Outcomes research, as defined by the Agency for Healthcare and Research Quality (AHRQ), is the investigation and comparison of patient experiences following treatment of a disease or injury.[1] The growing incidence, prevalence, and economic burden of any given disease stimulate outcomes research to streamline health care toward more efficient and effective practices. Its goal is to evaluate the structure of our health care system and its processes from patient events and experiences that are of interest to patients, providers, policy makers, and third-party payers.[2] Patient experience is defined broadly, and can range from mortality to quality of life (**Table 1**).[3] The analysis of these outcomes is essential to guide clinical decision making and determine the best practices for those diseases and conditions that confer a great burden on our society.

Rheumatoid arthritis (RA) is the most common inflammatory joint disease and causes substantial disability and premature death for more than 1 million individuals in the United States.[4] Progressive and persistent inflammation of the synovial tissue causes early joint destruction, most frequently in the hand.[5] RA typically presents in young adulthood, and has a profound effect on an individual's ability to attend to their activities of daily living, vocational productivity, and quality of life. On a societal level, the effect of these lost wages and expensive medical therapies consume approximately $3.6 billion per year.[6,7] Furthermore, patients with the most severe manifestations of RA account for most of the health care expenditure related to medical and surgical therapies.[8]

Although there is no cure available, multiple surgical options are available to prevent the progression of joint destruction, including distal ulna resection and tenosynovectomy, and to reconstruct joints destroyed by RA, including joint arthrodesis or arthroplasty.[9] Although early aggressive treatment can slow or halt the progression of disease, medical therapies remain extremely expensive, and great controversy among clinicians exists regarding the effectiveness and timing of surgical intervention.[5,10] The current treatment of rheumatoid hand disease is marked by wide variations in clinical practice, limited data from small nonrandomized studies, and differing perspectives on the effectiveness of therapy from clinicians. In recent years, there has been a growing interest in the hand surgery specialty to apply the principles of outcomes research to better serve patients with RA. This review focuses on the variations in care that underscore our current treatment, the scope of outcomes assessment tools, and the current state of outcomes research in rheumatoid hand disease.

VARIATION IN CARE FOR RHEUMATOID HAND DISEASE

Variations in health care arise when there is no accepted standard of care for a given clinical problem, and when controversy and uncertainty exist regarding the best treatment option.

Supported in part by a Midcareer Investigator Award in Patient-Oriented Research (K24 AR053120) from the National Institute of Arthritis and Musculoskeletal and Skin Diseases (to Dr Kevin C. Chung).
Financial disclosures and conflicts of interest: the authors have nothing to disclose.
Section of Plastic Surgery, Department of Surgery, The University of Michigan Medical School, 1500 East Medical Center Drive, 2130 Taubman Center, SPC 5340, Ann Arbor, MI 48109-5340, USA
* Corresponding author.
E-mail address: kecchung@umich.edu

Table 1
Examples of health outcomes applicable to hand surgery

Measure	Example
Mortality	30-day postoperative mortality
Physiologic measures	Joint range of motion
Clinical events	Wound infection
Symptoms	Pain
Functional measures	Quality of life score
Patient satisfaction	Consumer Assessment of Health Plans (CAHPs) survey

Variations are typically believed to be geographic, but can also be classified by the sociodemographic characteristics of patients and providers. Multiple factors can contribute to variations in care, including logistical considerations, such as patient access to care, the epidemiology of disease, clinician density in a geographic area, and economic stresses.[11–14] For rheumatoid hand disease, both geographic as well as sociodemographic variation in treatment practices have been described.

Globally, the treatment of rheumatoid hand disease varies by the economic status of a country, cultural factors, and the presence of other disease burdens. For example, in Germany, health care reimbursement is largely fee-for-service, and most patients with RA are cared for by primary care physicians. There is, therefore, an economic incentive to avoid referring patients with RA to specialists, as this could result in revenue loss. Conversely, the Dutch health care system is a capitated system, and it is likely more financially beneficial to shift the cost of caring for patients with RA to specialist providers.[15,16] In a recent qualitative analysis of rheumatoid hand disease globally, economically developed countries, such as the United States, France, and Japan, adopt aggressive RA treatment options. Conversely, in the developing world, there is a far greater health burden related to communicable disease, such as tuberculosis, dysentery, and human immunodeficiency virus (HIV)/AIDS, that far outweighs the burden of RA in these populations. In these settings, expensive and invasive treatments for rheumatoid hand disease are not a priority but a luxury.[17] Cultural differences and expectations influence treatment. For example, in China, there is much stronger emphasis and reliance on the

family structure to care for disabled family members and elders. This often dissuades patients from pursuing surgical intervention for RA hand deformities, because they may have adequate support from relatives and are able to keep up their self-care with this assistance. In the United States, many elderly people live independently because of the rising costs of assisted living. This, coupled with different family cultural expectations, may motivate patients with rheumatoid hand disease to seek medical and surgical treatment so that they are able to attend to their own needs.[16]

In the United States, wide variation exists in the rates of surgical procedures for rheumatoid hand disease by geography, patient age, and patient gender.[18] For example, a cross-sectional survey looking at the rates of joint fusion, tenosynovectomy, and arthroplasty revealed wide variation in the rates of these procedures by geographic location, irrespective of the number of hand surgeons, disease prevalence, or the sociodemographic profile of the region. Ninety percent of procedures were performed in urban areas, and with a difference in rates ranging from a factor of 9.4 for arthroplasty, 11.7 for arthrodesis, and 9.5 for tenosynovectomy procedures. Men are more likely to receive prophylactic surgical procedures and surgery at a younger age compared with women, who are more likely to receive end-stage reconstruction. The reasons behind these variations are unclear, but may relate to differing patient and physician perspectives. For example, physicians report that women are more likely to value hand appearance compared with men, and are more willing to undergo surgery compared with men. An analysis of patient perspectives reveals that women and men are equally willing to undergo surgery, and value hand appearance and function similarly.[19] Furthermore, pain and joint function are primary motivators for surgery compared with hand appearance.[20] Prior research has also demonstrated that hand surgeons and rheumatologists have contrasting views on the appropriateness and timing of surgery for rheumatoid hand disease. For example, rheumatologists are often skeptical of the efficacy of prophylactic and therapeutic surgery for RA, and prefer to treat patients pharmacologically. They may view the need for surgery as a failure or inadequacy of their treatment regimen. Rheumatologists believe that hand surgeons may be overly aggressive in their approach to patients, and inappropriately optimistic regarding the benefits of surgery.[21,22] Conversely, hand surgeons believe that patients are referred too late for surgery to prevent further joint destruction, and potentially lose the opportunity to reconstruct functional and aesthetically acceptable hands in RA hands with advanced deformities. Only half of the surgeons believe that there is high-quality research to support the usefulness of rheumatoid hand surgical procedures, and far fewer rheumatologists believe that there are high-quality data to affirm the value of surgical reconstruction. Both rheumatologists and surgeons believe that the other's knowledge of surgical options and outcomes is suboptimal, and overestimate their ability to communicate with one another. Less than 20% of hand surgeons and rheumatologists treat patients with RA in a multidisciplinary setting.[10] For all of these reasons, it is extremely difficult to build consensus between providers regarding the indications and timing of surgical intervention in rheumatoid hand disease, and to develop a multidisciplinary approach to patient care. These controversies underscore the importance of robust outcome studies with rigorous methodology to guide clinical decision making and optimize patient care.

OUTCOMES ASSESSMENT IN RHEUMATOID HAND DISEASE

There are multiple instruments designed to collect outcome data from patients with RA, but currently, there is no standard or ideal method to capture all relevant patient outcomes. **Table 2**[23–45] details selected methods for assessing patient outcomes in rheumatoid hand disease.

Objective measures of function include assessments of range of motion and power, anatomic deformity, and function. These measures range from simple bedside testing to complex batteries of tasks related to activities of daily living. The majority are simple to obtain during a clinical visit in an efficient manner. For example, measures of active and passive range of motion with flexion and extension, and grip and pinch strength, can be quickly obtained in the office, and followed over time.[23,24] Anatomic deformity can be assessed by clinical examination or serial radiographs. For example, the Hand Index uses measurements of the span and lateral height of the open and closed hand to create a standardized measure of deformity that can be used to follow and compare patients.[25] The Joint Alignment and Motion (JAM) score and the mechanical joint score can be used to define hand deformity and dysfunction at the bedside, but are subject to observer variation.[26,27] The Sharp Index uses standardized criteria on radiographs to document progression of disease.[28] More complex methods of objective testing include the Jebsen-Taylor test,

the Grip Ability Test, or the Arthritis Hand Function Test. These may provide a better assessment of difficulty with activities of daily living, but may not be well correlated with other important end points such as pain, aesthetics, and patient satisfaction. Overall, objective measures are advantageous in that they can be easily compared across studies, but are subject to observer variation. In addition, they do not capture the full extent of patient disability, such as pain and dissatisfaction. Many patients are able to retain excellent hand functioning despite deformity. Therefore, pain, joint instability, and exercise tolerance are more predictive of physical functioning and general health perception among patients with RA than clinical or radiologic joint appearance.[46–48]

Patient perception of health status is an essential component of outcomes assessment, and may be a better predictor of functional status and disability compared with objective measures.[49] However, patient self-assessment tools can be ineffective if they are lengthy, nonspecific, and/or cannot capture cultural differences between groups. Furthermore, they may not capture all elements of disability that are of interest to patients and investigators. Many instruments have been used to define patient-related outcomes in patients with RA, ranging from general quality of life to hand-specific surveys. General health assessment instruments, such as the visual analog scale (VAS), the SF-36 and its derivations, and the Health Assessment Questionnaire (HAQ), offer a global assessment of functioning.[38,50,51] The SF-36 is a well known and widely used measure of general quality of life and global functioning. However, it does not capture the amount of disability specifically related to RA or hand dysfunction.[37] Similarly, the VAS is easily completed by respondents, and has been modified to include a hand disability module validated for patients with RA.[39] The HAQ is widely used in studies comparing the effectiveness of different medical treatments for RA, but does not specifically address issues that may be more pertinent to postoperative outcomes. The Arthritis Impact Measurement Scales 2 questionnaire is a 45-item, self-administered outcomes tool designed to assess health status in patients with inflammatory arthritis and osteoarthritis. It is designed to provide a global self-reported assessment of patient health status. It has been widely used and well validated in patients with RA and can be used to capture specific quality of life outcomes in this population, including arm disability.[40]

Hand-specific outcome assessment tools can provide greater insight into the nuances of rheumatoid hand disability. The Australian Canadian

Table 2
Selected outcomes assessment tools for measuring rheumatoid hand outcomes

Name	Characteristics	Extremities Assessed	Time
Objective Measurements and Functional Testing			
Range of motion[23]	Measured with a geniometer to determine active and passive range of motion with flexion and extension, and abduction and adduction. Can also determine hyperextension, extension lag, and flexion block	Single joint or total finger measurements	<1 min
Grip and pinch strength[24]	Grip: measured with a dynamometer or sphygmomanometer to determine dysfunction. Difficult to determine muscle, tendon dysfunction, or joint instability in isolation. Can measure standard dynamic grip strength, time to achieve 95% of maximum grip strength, maximum power outputs Pinch: tip, tripod, and lateral pinch can be measured using pinch gauge instruments	Each hand assessed separately	<5 min
The Hand Index[25]	Span and lateral height of the open and closed hand are measured and standardized by the following formula: open hand span − closed hand span/lateral height of the hand	Each hand assessed separately	<5 min
The Joint Alignment and Motion Score[26]	5-point scale based on the % of normal range of motion and joint alignment	Each hand assessed separately	5 min
Mechanical Joint Score[27]	Clinical joint appearance rated on a scale of 0−3 based on observer appreciation of deformity	Each hand assessed separately	5 min
The Sharp Index[28]	Joint destruction assessed by radiographs and scored	Each hand assessed separately	Variable
Sequential Occupational Dexterity Assessment[29]	12 ADL-related tasks are used to assess ability to complete tasks (clinician rated), pain (patient rated), and function (patient rated). Quality of performance, independent of time, is measured	Both hands: 4 unilateral and 8 bilateral tests	Variable
Keitel Hand Functional Index[30,31]	Uses 24 movement tests to measure upper extremity function. Can assess the thumb, fingers and wrist separately	Each hand assessed separately	1 min
Jebsen-Taylor Test[32]	Standardized and objective assessment of hand functioning with 7 tasks: (1) writing a short sentence, (2) turning over cards, (3) picking up small objects and placing them in a container, (4) simulated feeding, (5) moving large empty cans, (6) moving a large weighted can, and (7) picking up checkers	Each hand assessed separately	15 min
Purdue peg board[33]	Times the ability of the individual to place prefabricated pins in holes of a pegboard, and assemble pins, washers, and collars in each hole	Each hand assessed separately, then together	15 min

Instrument	Description	Assessment	Time
Grip Ability Test[34,35]	Measures applied grip strength through 3 tasks: (1) putting a flexigrip stocking over the nondominant hand, (2) putting a paper clip on an envelope, and (3) pouring water from a jug	Each hand assessed separately	5 min
Arthritis Hand Function Test[36]	11-item test measuring grip and pinch strength, dexterity (each hand and applied), and strength	Each hand assessed separately and together	Variable
Self-assessment Instruments			
SF-36[37]	36-item survey that determines functional health and well-being along 8 scales generally divided into physical and mental health	Symptoms related to upper extremity disability not specifically assessed	5–10 min
Health Assessment Questionnaire (HAQ)[38]	20 items. Measures global functioning and health status in patients with arthritis (all types) along the following domains: (1) disability, (2) discomfort and pain, (3) drug side effects (toxicity), and (4) dollar costs. The disability index is most commonly used, and consists of 20 items measuring 8 subscales: eating, walking, rising, hygiene, activities, grip, dressing, reach	Symptoms related to upper extremity disability not specifically assessed	20 min
VAS-RA and VAS-hand[39]	2 questions query patients on the extent of disability related to RA, and rheumatoid hand disease, rated on a 10-point horizontal visual analog scale	Extremities assessed simultaneously	<1 min
Arthritis Impact Measurement Scales (AIMS)[40]	45 items that measure arthritis-specific health status along 9 domains including mobility, physical activity, dexterity, household activities, ADLs, anxiety, depression, social activity, and pain	Extremities assessed simultaneously	20 min
Australian/Canadian Osteoarthritis Hand Index[41]	15 items designed to measure 3 domains: pain, function, and stiffness	Bilateral	7 min
Disabilities of the Arm and Shoulder questionnaire[42]	30 items relating to function, ability to complete ADLs, social limitations, pain, sleep disturbance, and self-consciousness. Also includes a separate module for athletes and musicians	Single, entire upper extremity assessed as a unit	7 min
Michigan Hand Questionnaire[43]	37 items designed to measure hand performance along 6 domains: function, activities of daily living, pain, work performance, aesthetics, and satisfaction	Both assessed separately. Controls for hand dominance and diseased hand	15 min
Patient-related wrist evaluation[44]	15 items designed to measure pain and functional disability, specific to hand and wrist disability	Left and right assessed separately	5 min
Cochin Rheumatoid Hand Disability Scale[45]	RA-specific instrument with 18 items aimed at assessing ability to complete ADLs including the following 5 categories: (1) kitchen, (2) dressing, (3) hygiene, (4) office, and (5) others	Left and right assessed separately	3 min

Abbreviation: ADL, activity of daily life.

Osteoarthritis Hand Index is a 15-item self-assessment tool designed to measure the status of hand function with respect to pain, function, and stiffness, and has been validated against other measures in rheumatoid hand disease.[41] The Disability of the Arm, Shoulder, and Hand (DASH) questionnaire has been widely used to study hand disability, and incorporates a module for musicians and athletes. However, it has not been specifically validated in RA, and does not distinguish between the right and left upper extremity, and specific location of the upper extremity disability (fingers, hand, wrist, elbow, or shoulder).[42] The Michigan Hand Outcomes (MHQ) is a 37-item self-assessment instrument that measures disability along 6 domains: function, activities of daily living, pain, hand appearance, patient satisfaction, and work disability. It has been widely used to study a variety of acute and chronic disease conditions, and has been validated in patients with RA.[43,52–60] The Patient Related Wrist Evaluation is a 15-item instrument that measures pain and disability of the wrist, but does not include measures of hand appearance, and it may be difficult to elucidate the extent of patient disability related to the hand and phalanges.[44] The Cochin Rheumatoid Hand Disability scale is an 18-item scale that determines disability related to activities of daily living. It is quick to complete and responsive to clinical change, but does not specify disability by right or left extremity.[44,45,61,62]

There are an enormous number of surveys, tests, and scales with which disability caused by RA can be determined, and currently there is no standard measure.[63,64] Therefore, it is important for investigators to choose those tools that have been validated in RA populations, are specific to the outcome of interest, and can be combined with other methods to comprehensively and accurately capture patient outcomes.

CURRENT STATE OF OUTCOMES RESEARCH IN RHEUMATOID HAND DISEASE AND FUTURE DIRECTIONS

Previous studies regarding surgical treatment options for rheumatoid hand disease have been marked by small sample size, heterogeneous outcome measurements, and retrospective case series study design. A brief description of the challenges in rheumatoid hand outcomes research is displayed in **Table 3**. Specifically, these include small single-center studies with case series design with heterogeneous outcome measures. Such limitations have contributed to the variation in care seen with surgical treatment as providers cannot be clearly guided to best treatment strategies by ineffective evidence.[65] Therefore, it is critical to redirect our current research efforts to obtain clinically relevant and robust studies to guide clinical decision making. Several different study methodologies in outcomes research offer new strategies to overcome these challenges.

Qualitative Research

Qualitative research has been defined as "An inquiry process of understanding … that explore[s] a social or human problem. The researcher builds a complex, holistic picture, analyzes words, reports detailed views of informants, and conducts the study in a natural setting."[66] Qualitative research is powerful in that it can capture phenomena not assessed with more quantitative methods, as it is not constrained by investigator-selected criteria or questions. Nonetheless, it remains a frequently

Table 3
Challenges to outcomes research in rheumatoid hand disease and potential strategies for improvement

Challenges in Outcomes Research	Strategies for Improvement
Single-center studies/care series	Multidisciplinary, multicenter collaborative studies
Heterogeneous outcomes measurements	Standardized survey instruments to collect pertinent outcomes data, qualitative studies to elucidate outcomes relevant to patients
Small study sample size	Systematic/comparative effectiveness reviews, decision analysis (eg, Markov modeling)
Heterogeneous study samples	Rigorous inclusion criteria
Difficulty randomizing patients to surgical interventions	Decision analysis with hypothetical scenarios, cohort or case-control study design incorporating control groups
Retrospective studies	Prospective multicenter studies

underutilized methodology in surgical research. However, several qualitative studies have detailed RA patient outcomes using qualitative design methods with interesting and clinically relevant findings. For example, Mancuso and colleagues[67] interviewed 22 patients with RA to identify the challenges of patients in their workplace. These investigators were able to identify several barriers that may be easily predicted, such as fatigue and ability to write. In addition, they also determined other important barriers, such as mental attitude and difficulty with commuting, and strategies to overcome these, such as career choices and using ancillary services that may not have been captured by quantitative methods or standardized outcomes assessment tools. Qualitative research can also be used for the development and validation of standardized instruments. For example, the MHQ was developed using qualitative survey methods incorporating feedback from hand therapists, patients, and hand surgeons to identify important domains in rheumatoid hand disease outcomes.[43] Furthermore, Tammaru and colleagues[68] used qualitative methods to determine if a previously validated quality-of-life (QOL) tool would be applicable to diverse populations. These investigators used semi-structured interviews with RA patients and compared the results against a standardized QOL survey. The investigators identified several areas of concern for those specific patients not captured by the standardized instrument. Qualitative research can be used to identify strategies for improvement in practice. For example, Haugli and colleagues[69] conducted interviews with 26 patients with inflammatory arthritis and other noninflammatory conditions. Compared with patients with noninflammatory disorders, patients with RA and other inflammatory arthritis conditions felt depersonalized as a result of their diagnosis and that their pain may not be recognized fully. Although qualitative research has not been widely adopted to study patient outcomes in rheumatoid hand disease, it has the potential to offer rich and unique data that can direct clinicians and researchers toward important clinical outcomes.

Systematic Reviews

Systematic reviews are comprehensive summaries of the existing literature regarding a specific topic of interest, and are particularly useful to answer questions in scenarios in which the existing literature primarily consists of multiple nonrandomized case series.[70] Such reviews not only contain a description of the findings in the collection of studies but can also incorporate analysis and quantitative pooling of data, or a meta-analysis.

AHRQ has recently modified the description of systematic reviews to comparative effectiveness reviews, which detail the relative benefits and drawbacks of treatment options for a clinical problem, rather than attempt to answer a single question. The biggest strength of such reviews is that they can be used to synthesize and consolidate several data for clinical problems for which it is prohibitively difficult to conduct a large multicenter study.[71] In this way, they can provide strong evidence to identify the best treatment options for patients. For example, controversy exists regarding the benefits of wrist arthroplasty over total wrist fusion for rheumatoid wrist disease. Despite offering the possibility of greater wrist range of motion, wrist arthroplasty is more technically challenging, costly, and time consuming compared with total wrist fusion. A recent systematic review pooled 20 studies and more than 800 procedures looking at outcomes after both procedures. In this review, functional outcomes and range of motion after wrist fusion were similar compared with arthroplasty.[72] Such data can be used to change practice patterns and direct surgeons to performing more efficient and safer care.

Furthermore, systematic reviews can highlight areas of uncertainty to focus future research. For example, Ghattas and colleagues[73] conducted a systematic review to summarize the role of surgery in rheumatoid hand disease. Out of 196 studies identified, only 5 were randomized trials, and most were observational studies. Although these studies were too heterogeneous for meta-analysis, this review identified important limitations in the current literature, and possibilities for change such as having control groups in the study design and recruiting as homogeneous patient sample as possible. Outcomes to be measured should ideally be uniform between medical and surgical therapies, and focus on those significant to the patient experience, such as pain and ability to complete activities of daily living. Such observations are true even with respect to the medical treatment of rheumatoid hand disease. For example, a systematic review looking at the use of patient-reported outcome measures in the RA literature found heterogeneous outcomes in the studies reviewed. Only function, patient global assessment of well-being, and stiffness were consistently reported in more than 25% of articles.[50] Conversely, other outcomes, such as fatigue, psychological status, and coping were not widely reported, although are clinically relevant to patients. Systematic reviews can be an essential strategy to synthesize our current knowledge, obtain summary statistics when obtaining large sample sizes is not feasible, and identify new areas of study in rheumatoid hand disease.

Decision Analysis

When there is a paucity of rigorous clinical data, the decision for treatment is often made based on anecdotal experiences and patient/surgeon preferences. However, decision analysis is an important technique by which treatment options can be compared, and have been successfully used in rheumatoid hand disease.[74–76] Decision analysis assigns ratings or values to a specific patient outcome or health state. It also allows for dissimilar outcomes and procedures to be compared using standardized measures, such as cost comparisons relative to quality-adjusted life-years. Decision analysis can be used to better understand the motivations and discrepancies behind why some physicians favor certain treatments more than others. For example, when presented with scenarios regarding nonoperative management, total wrist arthroplasty, and arthrodesis for rheumatoid wrist disease, both rheumatologists and hand surgeons report that life with the manifestations of rheumatoid wrist disease is worth approximately half of a life with a normal wrist.[76,77] However, there is no change between arthroplasty and arthrodesis among surgeons, which may explain why many surgeons have failed to adopt arthroplasty into their practice for rheumatoid wrist disease. Patients also rated life with rheumatoid wrist disease extremely unfavorably, and much lower than physicians ratings.[78] This may indicate that clinicians underestimate the devastating effect rheumatoid hand disease has on quality of life, and may signal a need to refer patients earlier for surgical consultation. As displayed in this example, decision analysis can uncover mechanisms that underlie observed variations in care and can highlight patient and provider motivations for deciding between treatment options.

Prospective Studies

For all methodologies, prospective comparative studies offer a robust study design and the soundest evidence for determining appropriate treatment options. However, they are challenging for those diseases that are relatively rare, as it can be expensive and logistically difficult to accrue a large enough sample size to discern statistically and clinically significant differences in treatment options. Furthermore, it is difficult to randomize patients to surgical therapy for ethical reasons and patient preference. Nonetheless, several groups have developed prospective cohorts to follow patients with RA over time for many study purposes.

One of the largest prospective cohorts of patients with RA was brought together by Japanese investigators through the Institute of Rheumatology, Rheumatoid Arthritis (IORRA) study. Using data collected prospectively since 2000, these investigators have been able to analyze trends in surgical therapy, cost of treatment, and the development of adverse conditions related to immunomodulatory therapies.[79–86] In Sweden, several large, nationally based registries have been established that have studied the efficacy, safety, and long-term sequelae of medical therapies for RA.[87] Such studies are useful to describe chronologic trends in disease and treatment patterns, and can provide important information regarding the long-term durability and effectiveness of a given surgical procedure. However, they are limited by the end points selected by the investigators, the ability to maintain patient follow-up, and the availability of control groups for comparison. Furthermore, data collection can be challenging in large health care–based or national registries because they may not capture important variables related to the process or structure of care that may be relevant to patient outcomes. Regardless of these limitations, large prospective studies represent a critical strategy for obtaining rigorous outcome measures in rheumatoid hand disease.

Prospective studies are challenging for relatively rare diseases such as RA to achieve adequate samples size to identify significant findings. A multicenter, collaborative approach can not only easily increase sample size but also change the sociodemographic composition of the study population to improve generalizability. For example, a multicenter trial at the University of Michigan (Ann Arbor, MI, USA), Curtis National Hand Center (Baltimore, MD, USA), and the Pulvertaft Hand Center (Derby, England) has followed patients with rheumatoid hand disease prospectively to determine the efficacy of silicone metacarpophalangeal arthroplasty (SMPA).[88] Because randomization is difficult in this clinical setting, the surgical group included patients who chose to undergo SMPA, and the control group included patients who were managed medically. Both the surgical group and the control group were equally eligible for surgery based on the inclusion criteria to allow for a homogenous patient population. In order to assess patient outcomes after surgery, objective measures of hand functioning were obtained, including range of motion, extensor lag, ulnar drift, and Jebsen-Taylor test score.[89] Patient-reported outcomes were obtained using the MHQ and the AIMS2 survey. For example, at 1-year follow-up, patients with RA with poor functioning benefit from SMPA, based on both objective and patient self-assessment scores. Furthermore, even patients with severe RA deformity based on severe ulnar drift or extension lag benefitted similarly to patients with less severe deformity when undergoing SMPA.[53,90] These findings are important as these patients may previously have been deemed too diseased for surgical intervention. Not all measures improved equally. For example, although MHQ scores, ulnar deviation, and extension lag improved, there was no change in AIMS2 scores, grip, or pinch strength. Therefore, it is important to use a complement of self-assessment and objective testing to fully describe patient outcomes. Such studies that have a diverse population, prospective study design, and explicit inclusion and exclusion criteria represent the best evidence for surgical therapy for rheumatoid hand disease.

SUMMARY

Given the complex, fragile, and dynamic nature of our current health care economy, it is imperative that current research efforts and funding be directed toward identifying those practices that most efficiently and effectively benefit patients. Outcomes research plays a pivotal role as the foundation for understanding the quality of health care that is delivered, and how to optimize this care. RA presents a unique research challenge as it afflicts a young productive population, but is rare enough that accruing sufficient patient samples in a prospective manner can be expensive and challenging. However, outcomes research can provide rigorous methodology and robust data that can build consensus regarding the best treatment strategies for rheumatoid hand disease and yield high-quality efficient health care for our patients.

REFERENCES

1. The outcome of outcomes research at AHCPR: final report. Available at: http://www.ahrq.gov/clinic/out2res/. Accessed October 1, 2010.
2. Donabedian A. The quality of care. How can it be assessed? JAMA 1988;260:1743–8.
3. Clancy CM, Eisenberg JM. Outcomes research: measuring the end results of health care. Science 1998;282:245–6.
4. Helmick CG, Felson DT, Lawrence RC, et al. Estimates of the prevalence of arthritis and other rheumatic conditions in the United States. Part I. Arthritis Rheum 2008;58:15–25.
5. O'Dell JR. Therapeutic strategies for rheumatoid arthritis. N Engl J Med 2004;350:2591–602.
6. Sherrer YS, Bloch DA, Mitchell DM, et al. The development of disability in rheumatoid arthritis. Arthritis Rheum 1986;29:494–500.
7. Ward MM, Javitz HS, Yelin EH. The direct cost of rheumatoid arthritis. Value Health 2000;3:243–52.
8. Rat AC, Boissier MC. Rheumatoid arthritis: direct and indirect costs. Joint Bone Spine 2004;71:518–24.
9. Chung KC, Kotsis SV. Outcomes of hand surgery in the patient with rheumatoid arthritis. Curr Opin Rheumatol 2010;22:336–41.
10. Alderman AK, Chung KC, Kim HM, et al. Effectiveness of rheumatoid hand surgery: contrasting perceptions of hand surgeons and rheumatologists. J Hand Surg Am 2003;28:3–11 [discussion: 2–3].
11. McPherson K, Wennberg JE, Hovind OB, et al. Small-area variations in the use of common surgical procedures: an international comparison of New England, England, and Norway. N Engl J Med 1982;307:1310–4.
12. Wennberg JE. Understanding geographic variations in health care delivery. N Engl J Med 1999;340:52–3.
13. Welch WP, Miller ME, Welch HG, et al. Geographic variation in expenditures for physicians' services in the United States. N Engl J Med 1993;328:621–7.
14. Chung KC, Kotsis SV, Fox DA, et al. Differences between the United States and the United Kingdom in the treatment of rheumatoid arthritis: analyses from a hand arthroplasty trial. Clin Rheumatol 2010;29:363–7.
15. Waltz M. The disease process and utilization of health services in rheumatoid arthritis: the relative contributions of various markers of disease severity in explaining consumption patterns. Arthritis Care Res 2000;13:74–88.
16. Kotsis SV, Chung KC. A qualitative assessment of rheumatoid hand surgery in various regions of the world. J Hand Surg Am 2005;30:649–57.
17. Kalla AA, Tikly M. Rheumatoid arthritis in the developing world. Best Pract Res Clin Rheumatol 2003;17:863–75.
18. Alderman AK, Chung KC, Demonner S, et al. The rheumatoid hand: a predictable disease with unpredictable surgical practice patterns. Arthritis Rheum 2002;47:537–42.
19. Alderman AK, Arora AS, Kuhn L, et al. An analysis of women's and men's surgical priorities and willingness to have rheumatoid hand surgery. J Hand Surg Am 2006;31:1447–53.
20. Chung KC, Kotsis SV, Kim HM, et al. Reasons why rheumatoid arthritis patients seek surgical treatment for hand deformities. J Hand Surg Am 2006;31:289–94.

21. Alderman AK, Ubel PA, Kim HM, et al. Surgical management of the rheumatoid hand: consensus and controversy among rheumatologists and hand surgeons. J Rheumatol 2003;30:1464–72.

22. Glickel SZ. Commentary: effectiveness of rheumatoid hand surgery. J Hand Surg 2003;28:12–3.

23. Eberhardt KB, Svensson B, Mortiz U. Functional assessment of early rheumatoid arthritis. Br J Rheumatol 1988;27:364–71.

24. Myers DB, Grennan DM, Palmer DG. Hand grip function in patients with rheumatoid arthritis. Arch Phys Med Rehabil 1980;61:369–73.

25. Highton J, Markham V, Doyle TC, et al. Clinical characteristics of an anatomical hand index measured in patients with rheumatoid arthritis as a potential outcome measure. Rheumatology (Oxford) 2005; 44:651–5.

26. Spiegel TM, Spiegel JS, Paulus HE. The Joint Alignment and Motion scale: a simple measure of joint deformity in patients with rheumatoid arthritis. J Rheumatol 1987;14:887–92.

27. Johnson AH, Hassell AB, Jones PW, et al. The mechanical joint score: a new clinical index of joint damage in rheumatoid arthritis. Rheumatology (Oxford) 2002;41:189–95.

28. Sharp JT. Scoring radiographic abnormalities in rheumatoid arthritis. J Rheumatol 1989;16:568–9.

29. van Lankveld WG, Graff MJ, van 't Pad Bosch PJ. The Short Version of the Sequential Occupational Dexterity Assessment based on individual tasks' sensitivity to change. Arthritis Care Res 1999;12: 417–24.

30. Kalla AA, Kotze TJ, Meyers OL, et al. Clinical assessment of disease activity in rheumatoid arthritis: evaluation of a functional test. Ann Rheum Dis 1988;47:773–9.

31. Kalla AA, Smith PR, Brown GM, et al. Responsiveness of Keitel functional index compared with laboratory measures of disease activity in rheumatoid arthritis. Br J Rheumatol 1995;34:141–9.

32. Jebsen RH, Taylor N, Trieschmann RB, et al. An objective and standardized test of hand function. Arch Phys Med Rehabil 1969;50:311–9.

33. Hardin M. Assessment of hand function and fine motor coordination in the geriatric population. Top Geriatr Rehabil 2002;18:18–27.

34. Dellhag B, Bjelle A. A grip ability test for use in rheumatology practice. J Rheumatol 1995;22:1559–65.

35. Dellhag B, Bjelle A. A five-year followup of hand function and activities of daily living in rheumatoid arthritis patients. Arthritis Care Res 1999;12:33–41.

36. Backman C, Mackie H, Harris J. Arthritis Hand Function Test: development of a standardized assessment tool. Occup Ther J Res 1991;11:245–56.

37. Talamo J, Frater A, Gallivan S, et al. Use of the short form 36 (SF36) for health status measurement in rheumatoid arthritis. Br J Rheumatol 1997;36:463–9.

38. Boers M, Felson DT. Clinical measures in rheumatoid arthritis: which are most useful in assessing patients? J Rheumatol 1994;21:1773–4.

39. Massy-Westropp N, Ahern M, Krishnan J. A visual analogue scale for assessment of the impact of rheumatoid arthritis in the hand: validity and repeatability. J Hand Ther 2005;18:30–3.

40. Meenan RF, Mason JH, Anderson JJ, et al. AIMS2. The content and properties of a revised and expanded Arthritis Impact Measurement Scales Health Status Questionnaire. Arthritis Rheum 1992; 35:1–10.

41. Massy-Westropp N, Krishnan J, Ahern M. Comparing the AUSCAN Osteoarthritis Hand Index, Michigan Hand Outcomes Questionnaire, and Sequential Occupational Dexterity Assessment for patients with rheumatoid arthritis. J Rheumatol 2004;31:1996–2001.

42. Beaton DE, Katz JN, Fossel AH, et al. Measuring the whole or the parts? Validity, reliability, and responsiveness of the disabilities of the arm, shoulder and hand outcome measure in different regions of the upper extremity. J Hand Ther 2001;14:128–46.

43. Chung KC, Pillsbury MS, Walters MR, et al. Reliability and validity testing of the Michigan Hand Outcomes Questionnaire. J Hand Surg Am 1998; 23:575–87.

44. MacDermid JC, Turgeon T, Richards RS, et al. Patient rating of wrist pain and disability: a reliable and valid measurement tool. J Orthop Trauma 1998;12:577–86.

45. Duruoz MT, Poiraudeau S, Fermanian J, et al. Development and validation of a rheumatoid hand functional disability scale that assesses functional handicap. J Rheumatol 1996;23:1167–72.

46. Yazici Y, Sokka T, Pincus T. Radiographic measures to assess patients with rheumatoid arthritis: advantages and limitations. Rheum Dis Clin North Am 2009;35:723–9, vi.

47. Eurenius E, Brodin N, Lindblad S, et al. Predicting physical activity and general health perception among patients with rheumatoid arthritis. J Rheumatol 2007;34:10–5.

48. Sears ED, Chung KC. Validity and responsiveness of the Jebsen-Taylor hand function test. J Hand Surg Am 2009;35(1):30–7.

49. Pincus T, Yazici Y, Bergman MJ. Patient questionnaires in rheumatoid arthritis: advantages and limitations as a quantitative, standardized scientific medical history. Rheum Dis Clin North Am 2009;35: 735–43, vii.

50. Kalyoncu U, Dougados M, Daures JP, et al. Reporting of patient-reported outcomes in recent trials in rheumatoid arthritis: a systematic literature review. Ann Rheum Dis 2009;68:183–90.

51. Boers M, Tugwell P, Felson DT, et al. World Health Organization and International League of

Associations for Rheumatology core endpoints for symptom modifying antirheumatic drugs in rheumatoid arthritis clinical trials. J Rheumatol Suppl 1994; 41:86–9.

52. Chang EY, Chung KC. Outcomes of trapeziectomy with a modified abductor pollicis longus suspension arthroplasty for the treatment of thumb carpometacarpal joint osteoarthritis. Plast Reconstr Surg 2008;122:505–15.

53. Chung KC, Burke FD, Wilgis EF, et al. A prospective study comparing outcomes after reconstruction in rheumatoid arthritis patients with severe ulnar drift deformities. Plast Reconstr Surg 2009;123: 1769–77.

54. Herweijer H, Dijkstra PU, Nicolai JP, et al. Postoperative hand therapy in Dupuytren's disease. Disabil Rehabil 2007;29:1736–41.

55. Chung KC, Ram AN, Shauver MJ. Outcomes of pyrolytic carbon arthroplasty for the proximal interphalangeal joint. Plast Reconstr Surg 2009;123: 1521–32.

56. Chung KC, Kotsis SV, Kim HM. Predictors of functional outcomes after surgical treatment of distal radius fractures. J Hand Surg Am 2007;32:76–83.

57. McMillan CR, Binhammer PA. Which outcome measure is the best? Evaluating responsiveness of the disabilities of the arm, shoulder, and hand questionnaire, the Michigan Hand Questionnaire and the patient-specific functional scale following hand and wrist surgery. Hand (N Y) 2009;4:311–8.

58. Klein RD, Kotsis SV, Chung KC. Open carpal tunnel release using a 1-centimeter incision: technique and outcomes for 104 patients. Plast Reconstr Surg 2003;111:1616–22.

59. Chung KC, Watt AJ, Kotsis SV. A prospective outcomes study of four-corner wrist arthrodesis using a circular limited wrist fusion plate for stage II scapholunate advanced collapse wrist deformity. Plast Reconstr Surg 2006;118:433–42.

60. Waljee JF, Chung KC, Kim HM, et al. The validity and responsiveness of the Michigan Hand Questionnaire (MHQ) in patients with rheumatoid arthritis: a multicenter, international study. Arthritis Care Res 2010; 62:1567–77.

61. Poiraudeau S, Lefevre-Colau MM, Fermanian J, et al. The ability of the Cochin rheumatoid arthritis hand functional scale to detect change during the course of disease. Arthritis Care Res 2000;13: 296–303.

62. Lefevre-Colau MM, Poiraudeau S, Fermanian J, et al. Responsiveness of the Cochin rheumatoid hand disability scale after surgery. Rheumatology (Oxford) 2001;40:843–50.

63. Chung KC, Burns PB, Davis Sears E. Outcomes research in hand surgery: where have we been and where should we go? J Hand Surg Am 2006; 31:1373–9.

64. Bindra RR, Dias JJ, Heras-Palau C, et al. Assessing outcome after hand surgery: the current state. J Hand Surg Br 2003;28:289–94.

65. Alderman AK, Chung KC. Measuring outcomes in hand surgery. Clin Plast Surg 2008;35:239–50.

66. Creswell JW, editor. Research design: qualitative and quantitative approaches. Thousand Oaks (CA): Sage Publications; 1994.

67. Mancuso CA, Paget SA, Charlson ME. Adaptations made by rheumatoid arthritis patients to continue working: a pilot study of workplace challenges and successful adaptations. Arthritis Care Res 2000;13: 89–99.

68. Tammaru M, Strompl J, Maimets K, et al. The value of the qualitative method for adaptation of a disease-specific quality of life assessment instrument: the case of the Rheumatoid Arthritis Quality of Life Scale (RAQoL) in Estonia. Health Qual Life Outcomes 2004;2:69.

69. Haugli L, Strand E, Finset A. How do patients with rheumatic disease experience their relationship with their doctors? A qualitative study of experiences of stress and support in the doctor-patient relationship. Patient Educ Couns 2004;52:169–74.

70. Margaliot Z, Chung KC. Systematic reviews: a primer for plastic surgery research. Plast Reconstr Surg 2007;120:1834–41.

71. Slutsky J, Atkins D, Chang S, et al. AHRQ series paper 1: comparing medical interventions: AHRQ and the effective health-care program. J Clin Epidemiol 2010;63:481–3.

72. Cavaliere CM, Chung KC. A systematic review of total wrist arthroplasty compared with total wrist arthrodesis for rheumatoid arthritis. Plast Reconstr Surg 2008;122:813–25.

73. Ghattas L, Mascella F, Pomponio G. Hand surgery in rheumatoid arthritis: state of the art and suggestions for research. Rheumatology (Oxford) 2005;44:834–45.

74. Chen NC, Shauver MJ, Chung KC. A primer on use of decision analysis methodology in hand surgery. J Hand Surg Am 2009;34:983–90.

75. Birkmeyer JD, Birkmeyer NO. Decision analysis in surgery. Surgery 1996;120:7–15.

76. Cavaliere CM, Chung KC. Total wrist arthroplasty and total wrist arthrodesis in rheumatoid arthritis: a decision analysis from the hand surgeons' perspective. J Hand Surg Am 2008;33:1744–55, 55 e1–2.

77. Cavaliere CM, Oppenheimer AJ, Chung KC. Reconstructing the rheumatoid wrist: a utility analysis comparing total wrist fusion and total wrist arthroplasty from the perspectives of rheumatologists and hand surgeons. Hand 2009;5(1):9–18.

78. Cavaliere CM, Chung KC. A cost-utility analysis of nonsurgical management, total wrist arthroplasty, and total wrist arthrodesis in rheumatoid arthritis. J Hand Surg Am 2010;35. 379.e2–391.e2.

79. Momohara S, Ikari K, Mochizuki T. Declining use of synovectomy surgery for patients with rheumatoid arthritis in Japan. Ann Rheum Dis 2009;68(2): 291–2.

80. Tanaka E, Inoue E, Mannalithara A, et al. Medical care costs of patients with rheumatoid arthritis during the prebiologics period in Japan: a large prospective observational cohort study. Mod Rheumatol 2010;20:46–53.

81. Momohara S, Inoue E, Ikari K, et al. Risk factors for wrist surgery in rheumatoid arthritis. Clin Rheumatol 2008;27:1387–91.

82. da Silva E, Doran MF, Crowson CS, et al. Declining use of orthopedic surgery in patients with rheumatoid arthritis? Results of a long-term population-based assessment. Arthritis Rheum 2003;49(2): 216–20.

83. Ward MM. Decreases in rates of hospitalizations for manifestations of severe rheumatoid arthritis, 1983–2001. Arthritis Rheum 2004;50:1122–31.

84. Weiss RJ, Stark A, Wick MC, et al. Orthopedic surgery of the lower limbs in 49802 rheumatoid arthritis patients: results from the Swedish National Inpatient Registry during 1987–2001. Ann Rheum Dis 2006;65:335–41.

85. Fevang BT, Lie SA, Havelin LI, et al. Reduction in orthopedic surgery among patients with chronic inflammatory joint disease in Norway, 1004–2004. Arthritis Rheum 2004;57:529–32.

86. Yamanaka H, Inoue E, Singh G, et al. Improvement of disease activity of rheumatoid arthritis patients from 2000 to 2006 in a large observational cohort study IORRA in Japan. Mod Rheumatol 2007;17: 283–9.

87. van Vollenhoven RF, Askling J. Rheumatoid arthritis registries in Sweden. Clin Exp Rheumatol 2005;23: S195–200.

88. Chung KC, Kowalski CP, Myra Kim H, et al. Patient outcomes following Swanson silastic metacarpophalangeal joint arthroplasty in the rheumatoid hand: a systematic overview. J Rheumatol 2000;27: 1395–402.

89. Chung KC, Kotsis SV, Kim HM. A prospective outcomes study of Swanson metacarpophalangeal joint arthroplasty for the rheumatoid hand. J Hand Surg Am 2004;29:646–53.

90. Chung KC, Kotsis SV, Wilgis EF, et al. Outcomes of silicone arthroplasty for rheumatoid metacarpophalangeal joints stratified by fingers. J Hand Surg Am 2009;34:1647–52.

Index

Note: Page numbers of article titles are in **boldface** type.

Hand Clin 27 (2011) 127–130
doi:10.1016/S0749-0712(10)00107-1

Moving?

Make sure your subscription moves with you!

To notify us of your new address, find your **Clinics Account Number** (located on your mailing label above your name), and contact customer service at:

Email: journalscustomerservice-usa@elsevier.com

800-654-2452 (subscribers in the U.S. & Canada)
314-447-8871 (subscribers outside of the U.S. & Canada)

Fax number: 314-447-8029

Elsevier Health Sciences Division
Subscription Customer Service
3251 Riverport Lane
Maryland Heights, MO 63043

*To ensure uninterrupted delivery of your subscription, please notify us at least 4 weeks in advance of move.

Printed and bound by CPI Group (UK) Ltd, Croydon, CR0 4YY

03/10/2024

01040354-0005